Economics, Medicine and Health Care

We work with leading authors to develop the
strongest educational materials in economics,
medicine and health care, bringing cutting-edge thinking and best
learning practice to a global market.

Under a range of well-known imprints, including
Financial Times Prentice Hall, we craft high-quality print and
electronic publications which help readers to understand
and apply their content, whether studying or at work.

To find out more about the complete range of our
publishing, please visit us on the World Wide Web at:
www.pearsoned.co.uk

Economics, Medicine and Health Care

Third Edition

Gavin Mooney

Professor of Health Economics and Director of the
Social and Public Health Economics Research Group
(SPHERe), Curtin University, Perth, Australia; and
Visiting Professor, Aarhus University, Denmark

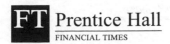 Prentice Hall
FINANCIAL TIMES

An imprint of **Pearson Education**
Harlow, England • London • New York • Boston • San Francisco • Toronto • Sydney • Singapore • Hong Kong
Tokyo • Seoul • Taipei • New Delhi • Cape Town • Madrid • Mexico City • Amsterdam • Munich • Paris • Milan

Pearson Education Limited
Edinburgh Gate
Harlow
Essex CM20 2JE
England

and Associated Companies throughout the world

Visit us on the World Wide Web at:
www.pearsoned.co.uk

First published 1986 by Wheatsheaf Books Limited
Second edition published 1992 by Prentice Hall Europe
Third edition published 2003 Pearson Education Limited

ISBN 0 273 65157 9

British Library Cataloguing-in-Publication Data
A catalogue record for this book is available from the British Library

10 9 8 7 6 5 4 3 2 1
08 07 06 05 04 03

Typeset in Times 10 on 12.5pt and Frutiger by 25
Printed in Great Britain by Henry Ling Ltd, at the Dorset Press, Dorchester, Dorset

The publisher's policy is to use paper manufactured from sustainable forests.

To faither

Contents

List of figures

List of tables

Preface to the first edition

In the process of writing this book I have been keenly aware of my need to learn more and more, particularly about health care. If economists are to succeed in persuading medical, nursing and other health care staff to pay more attention to our discipline, clearly we need to make some effort to understand the difficulties they face in their working environment. I have tried to do so. Certainly, I sympathise with them in the problems of resource allocation with which they have to grapple.

In that respect the book has benefited in being written from the medical campus of the University of Aberdeen, where I have been based since 1974. I would therefore like to express my gratitude to my medical colleagues, in particular Elizabeth Russell and Roy Weir, for their assistance and advice over the last few years.

A number of aspects of the book have benefited from discussions with fellow health economists outside Aberdeen. In particular, for their assistance and advice, I would like to thank Anita Alban, Yvonne Bally, Tony Culyer, Mike Drummond, Steve Engleman and Alan Williams.

It is, however, my long-suffering colleagues in the Health Economics Research Unit who deserve much of my gratitude. In particular, for their comments on various aspects of the book, I would like to thank Anne Ludbrook and Ali McGuire. Rochelle Coutts and Isabel Tudhope coped quite magnificently – as ever – with my handwriting in preparing the typescript, and I am grateful to them. In addition, I wish to thank an anonymous assessor for some very helpful suggestions.

I would also like to thank the many health service staff who have undertaken our correspondence courses in health economics. Some of the material has been drawn from that source and consequently benefited from their comments.

Finally, tak til Anita, Rikke og Johannes.

Gavin Mooney
University of Aberdeen, Aberdeen

Preface to the second edition

In revising this book I have been surprised at how much of what was originally written in 1984 and 1985 has survived reasonably intact. Of course things have changed and we have seen most recently the reforms of the NHS coming into place. We have also seen much more attention paid to quality adjusted life years (QALYs) than was the case in the mid-1980s. But there is a remarkable similarity in terms of the problems that health services still face.

Perhaps it is unrealistic to think that over just a few years there could be radical change. Yet, having been around health care for nearly 20 years, it is rather depressing to see how little does change. I remain convinced of the merits of trying to use economics to assist in the planning, financing and delivery of health care, and I believe there is a growing army of health service staff who are increasingly sharing that view. But there is no revolution. It is a gradual and slow process to get any change through. There is a conservatism to health services that is difficult to break through. Indeed, one of the clearest advantages of the NHS reforms is that they have been more successful in changing attitudes than any other change in recent years. Whether many of the good aspects of the reforms could have been achieved without quite so much of an upheaval remains a moot point. But the upheaval may have been necessary to get any sort of real change at all.

Beyond the acknowledgements in the preface to the first edition, I now want to add the names of those with whom my thought processes have developed over the last few years. They are many, but in particular I would want to recognise Anita Alban, Tony Culyer, Cam Donaldson, Jack Dowie, Mike Drummond, Ulrika Enemark, Karen Gerard, Matti Hakama, Jane Hall, Uffe Juul Jensen, Ivar Sønbø Kristiansen, Ali McGuire, Jan Abel Olsen and Alan Williams. Additionally, my thanks to two anonymous assessors who have helped me to clarify what I have been trying to say. I would also want to thank my wife Anita, and Rikke and Johannes, yet again for tolerating my absences and even more so my presences.

Gavin Mooney
Farum, Denmark

Preface to the third edition

Health services' policy-making and health economics seem, in the early years of this century, to be in the doldrums, neither quite knowing where they are going nor having any real wind in their sails. That is not necessarily a depressing observation. Too much action with too little thought was what the 1990s saw; too often me-too-ism as some new fashion resonated around the globe, or at least the developed globe. Some contemplation is needed. Some thinking through locally what the citizens of Denmark want from their health care system and what the citizens of South Africa want from theirs, and not assuming that health care goals are universal or that they are to be determined by policy-makers. It is not just goals that are culturally specific; so too are aspects of economic techniques. We may live in a globalising world but that does not mean we are all the same.

We are not even the same within countries: we do not have the same values; we do not necessarily share the same constructs of health or indeed of economics. Since writing the last edition of this book, I have become involved in research in Aboriginal health in Australia. That has changed much of my thinking, especially working with Shane Houston, Barbara Henry and Debby Woods. These Aboriginal people have taught me so much about the value base of health economics. Yet as I increasingly see economics as a branch of moral philosophy, I am comforted by the fact that my fellow Scot Adam Smith (not the right-wing market economist he is so often painted today) was Professor of Moral Philosophy when he wrote his *Wealth of Nations* in 1766.

I would hope that, in any contemplation on future health services policy-making, more and more policy-makers and planners, as well as those at the sharp end of health care, will see the merits of using and embracing health economics. Health economics can, I believe, supply important techniques and, more importantly, useful ideas. What it has been slow to do, although this is changing, is to accept any responsibility for engendering change. More and more (and especially among younger colleagues, such as Steve Jan and Virginia Wiseman), there is a recognition of a responsibility to seek change, not to try to dictate what that change might be but to examine not only what might be a better health care world but how barriers to change that the decision-makers might face might be reduced.

To the many students who have crawled over my materials for various courses over the years and made suggestions for improvements my thanks. To those who have said that you enjoyed the experience ... get a life!

My thanks go to many people who have shaped my thoughts in the last few years. My colleagues in SPHERe: Janet Dzator, Lucy Gilson, Barbara Henry, Shane Houston, Steve Jan, Di McIntyre, Glenn Salkeld, Alan Shiell, Virginia Wiseman and Debby Woods. Other colleagues who have contributed to my thoughts in all sorts of ways: Cam Donaldson, John Deeble, Karen Gerard, Uffe Juul Jensen, Ivar Sønbø Kristiansen, Miles Little, Robyn McDermott, Martha Nussbaum, Jan Abel Olsen, Aileen Plant, Tom Rice, Mandy Ryan and Ted Wilkes. My thanks, too, to Maggie Atherton, Jeanette Newcombe and Val Smith for keeping me (more or less) in line.

Gavin Mooney
Perth, Australia

Acknowledgements

We are grateful to the following for permission to reproduce copyright material:

Table 2.12 from Cost–benefit analysis of ambulance and rescue helicopters in Norway, in *Applied Health Economics and Health Policy*, Vol. 1 No. 2, Open Mind Journals Ltd (Elvick, R. 2002) adapted from Five hundred lifesaving interventions and their cost-effectiveness, in *Risk Analysis*, Vol. 15, Blackwell Publishing (Tengs, T.O., Adams, M.E. and Pliskin, J.E. 1995).

In some instances we have been unable to trace the owners of copyright material, and we would appreciate any information that would enable us to do so.

one

Introduction

> In the beginning, middle and end was, is and will be scarcity of resources.

From the standpoint of economics there is at least an appearance that much is wrong with health care. While an important part of this book, drawing attention to these issues is not its intent. Rather, the purpose is to provide the medical profession, other health care staff and maybe even some economists with some insights, from the perspective of the discipline of economics, into some of the issues currently facing many health services. It is hoped that such knowledge may help them to pursue better, more efficient and fairer delivery of health care.

It is a commonplace to say that the medical profession is held in a position of trust in society; it is equally a commonplace to state that the individual practitioner is held in a position of trust by the individual patient. A third relevant commonplace is to state that resources generally, and more specifically for health care, are scarce, with the consequence that not all wants or needs for health care can be met. What is not a commonplace – but ought to become one – is the fact that continued lack of general acceptance of the third point and the implications that flow from this lack may lead to an undermining of the trust in the first two with potentially serious consequences not only for the medical profession but for health care generally, and hence health. How do doctors make their decisions? What influences their behaviour? Research to answer these questions is growing but remains thin on the ground. What we do know, however, is that there are very substantial variations in medical practice which appear to imply that doctors are doing very different things when faced with similar patients. [1]

It is relatively easy to be critical of doctors because of their apparent ineffi-ciency. To understand better *why* they are inefficient is both more difficult and more important. Consequently, this book attempts not only to diagnose some of the ills of health care, some of which are indeed iatrogenic, but also to suggest some appropriate (i.e. the most cost-effective) treatments.

Our starting text is simply, 'In the beginning, middle and end was, is and will be scarcity of resources.' This is the essence of economics but unfortunately not – at least not sufficiently – of the science of medicine. It is around the concept of scarcity that this book revolves.

In the next chapter there is a brief introduction to economics and health eco-nomics that in no way does justice to the discipline but will provide a guide at minimum cost to doctors and others who have previously not encountered eco-nomics (at least not as a discipline – doctors inevitably encounter economics every day, even if they sometimes fail to appreciate the fact). How markets operate and the techniques of economic evaluation are also discussed in Chapter 2.

The third chapter considers a fundamental aspect of the whole debate about health care; that is, health care as a commodity (in the sense that, like cars, cakes and candelabra, it provides benefit, satisfaction and utility to consumers). It is a commodity, however, that in at least some respects is rather different from many, indeed most, other goods and services.

In the fourth chapter, the issue of quantifying health is outlined and the need for developing health status indices discussed. The use of quality adjusted life years (QALYs) is highlighted. That chapter also considers other possible outcomes from health care. This is followed in Chapter 5 by a debate on values in health care and especially whose values are relevant in health care, together with consideration of how economists have tackled the problem of valuing human life. Given that this is a task that is anathema to many health care professionals, it is important to ascer-tain why it cannot and should not be avoided.

This debate is continued in Chapter 6, where the concepts of demand and of need for health care are examined. This discussion is then set against the back-ground of the so-called 'agency relationship', a concept very familiar to and scarcely novel for doctors but discovered only relatively recently by economists. Here the various strands – scarcity, the nature of health care as an economic good, and values in health care – are brought together. However, this chapter does not offer any resolution of the tensions between these different facets and the actors playing the different roles.

Chapter 7 turns to some aspects of medical ethics, not only to make many readers feel more comfortable on more familiar territory but also to raise some slightly different questions both about and arising from medical ethics than is perhaps normally the case when such topics are debated. That then allows an indi-cation of the sort of conflict that apparently exists between economics and medi-cine. In reality, the conflict is more between, on the one hand, a rational acceptance of and approach to the issue of scarcity and, on the other, medical ethics (partly in principle but more so in practice). Indeed, in many ways it is the nature, source, problems and resolution of this conflict that are the central themes of this book.

Chapter 8 is about equity and the difficulties of defining it in practice. The link between ethics and equity is highlighted.

In Chapter 9 there is a discussion of various approaches to priority setting. This is one of the key ways in which economics can be of assistance to health care policy-makers. It is also an area that is ripe for improvement. Consequently this is debated at some length.

This is followed in Chapter 10 with some insights into financing and organisation of health care. While this is a massive topic, at least the key issues are identified and analysed. The rationale for different systems is discussed from the community's point of view. Essentially the arguments here are ideological.

What emerges from this is that the medical profession has attempted to retain, certainly individually but perhaps also collectively, an ideology or at least a modus operandi that is more appropriate in a market-oriented health care system. Indeed, it is suggested in Chapter 11 that in public health care systems medical doctors may have usurped some of the benefit of such systems not motivated by financial gain per se but rather as a means of defending their status. This chapter also points to a solution to some of the problems raised earlier in this book. The solution – essentially attempting to ensure that the objectives of the community qua community and those of the medical profession, both individually and collectively, become the same through the introduction of a new health care ethical code – is a simple one, at least in principle. Some mechanisms for providing the incentives for the medical profession to equate their objectives with the community's (or at least to behave as if this were the case) are presented. It is further emphasised that these mechanisms are wholly commensurate with, and may even enhance, most medical ethics, including the much-abused clinical freedom, provided medical ethics remains in its legitimate territory. Such demonstration should prevent besieged medical readers from labelling the process as unreasonable, unethical or impractical.

Notes

1. R.G. Evans, 'The dog in the night-time: medical practice variations of health policy' in *The Challenges of Medical Practice Variations*, eds T.F. Andersen and G.H. Mooney (Macmillan: London, 1990).

two

Economics and health economics

The social science – not a 'gay science' ... which finds the secret of this Universe in 'supply and demand' ... what we might call ... the dismal science.

Thomas Carlyle, 'On the Nigger Question' (1849)

2.1 Resource allocation problems

Economics has been defined by Samuelson as 'the study of how men and society end up choosing, with or without the use of money, to employ scarce productive resources that could have alternative uses, to produce various commodities and distribute them for consumption, now or in the future, among various people and groups in society. It analyses the costs and benefits of improving patterns of resource allocation.'[1]

Within this statement, which encompasses much more than many readers might have imagined, there are a number of important issues. In this chapter, rather briefly, I want to point out some of the main issues and exemplify them, where possible, in terms of health care or everyday life.

It would, however, be potentially misleading to venture into the process without first explaining that economics is a discipline, a recognised body of thought and not just a bag of tools. *Health economics* is the discipline of economics applied to the *topic* of health. Consequently, what health economists are doing when attempting to educate others – be they doctors, nurses, administrators, politicians, patients or the public generally – is primarily to try to change a way of thinking. It is not that economists would claim that their way of thinking is always 'superior'. It is unlikely to be the most helpful discipline in trying to solve a problem of nuclear physics or to run faster half-marathons. Yet there are economic questions surrounding these issues. How important is it to solve these problems? What proportion of society's scarce resources should be devoted to them? Why is it that as an individual I may devote more of my resources to the second (apparently trivial) problem than to the first? What is the most cost-effective solution to getting my time down – more training, better diet, fewer beers? Or maybe I would be better giving up running and taking up tennis or tiddlywinks instead?

There *are* economic issues here. They may well not be dominant, but there are few areas of life where economics does not come into play in some way or other. It seems difficult to believe, but it is nonetheless true, that economists have to try to persuade anyone that economics is important in health care – with some nations devoting over ten per cent of their total resources to health care (and considerably more to health), with technological advances appearing or developing much more rapidly than the ability and willingness to pay for them, with debates about the economic organisation of health care, questions about the role of prices and remuneration of manpower (e.g. doctors), and so on.

Thus, the issues of choice, as spelt out in Samuelson's definition, are relevant in health care. How much of society's scarce resources should be devoted to health, to health care? What priority should be given to the elderly vis-à-vis the mentally ill? What does 'giving priority' mean? Should more surgical patients be treated as day patients? When and where should that new hospital be built? Is prevention 'better' than cure, and, if so, for which diseases/conditions? What are the implications for the health service, for the community and for individual patients of introducing or increasing fees for consultation with general practitioners? What happens when we raise prescription charges?

Some of these questions appear more overtly economic than others; for example, when, as with the latter two issues, the question of money prices arises. In fact all of them involve choice about the use of scarce resources.

At this point, lest the reader begin to believe that they have already learned enough about the arrogance of economics, it is worth stressing that it is not suggested that economics alone can answer these questions. Indeed, economics will not even be the dominant discipline in trying to do so. There are essentially two points being made: (1) the occasions on which economics, particularly as a way of thinking, is likely to prove helpful are more frequent than most non-economists might expect; and (2) partly because of this, but also because of the methodological underpinning of all economics, an injection of such a way of thinking is likely to provide new and important insights that might otherwise have been overlooked.

Economics exists as a science of human behaviour for two simple reasons. First, there is a finite limit to the resources available to mankind as a whole, to any individual society, any organisation or, indeed, any individual. Second, as individuals and societies, it appears that to all intents and purposes our wants are insatiable. These two factors taken together mean that choice has to be exercised not only about what to do but also (and equally important) what to leave undone.

It follows from this that the concept of opportunity cost (which is rather different from the concept of cost that most non-economists understand) is central to economics. Strictly, it is the benefit foregone in the best alternative use of the resources. Opportunity cost thus entails sacrifice. Given that resources are scarce, if we decide to use them in one particular way, there is an opportunity foregone to obtain the benefits of using these resources in some other way. If I devote time (a scarce resource) to training for half-marathons, there is an opportunity cost involved in that I cannot use that same time to watch football, go to a concert or write books. If another computerised tomography (CT) scanner is bought, the costs and use represent foregone opportunities to provide benefits, from more geriatric beds, more health visiting or, in the end, more jogging or other forms of non-health care personal spending. Dr Paul *always* robs Dr, Mrs or Master Peita. As we shall see later, it is the *attempt* – inevitably forlorn – to ignore, bypass or overcome this basic law of economics that leads to frustration and inefficiency in the health care sector.

This concept of 'opportunity cost' encourages us to place monetary values on 'costs' that might not normally be seen as having pound signs in front of them, or indeed as costs at all. Thus, in the example of the use of time for training for half-marathons, the opportunity cost may be in measurable income foregone in not working. If this is the next best use of my time, then the amount of income foregone is a measure of the benefit I perceive I get from training. (The perception issue is important: if my running times do not improve, then I may realise that I would have been better off in writing than training. Nonetheless, I made the decision on the basis of my perception of the opportunity costs *at the time* I made the decision.)

Thus, in our private lives, albeit not necessarily wholly consciously, we attempt to maximise benefit from whatever resources we have at our disposal. This is essentially what efficiency is: getting the most out of the resources available. For example, some readers may have a penchant for avocados, as I do. Others may prefer oranges. Nonetheless, there is a limit to the number of avocados that I can or want to consume. At some stage, as I go on buying more and more avocado pears in a particular week, I will decide that I would rather have an orange than yet another avocado. Indeed, over a year it is likely that out of my budget for fruit I consume 100 avocados and 50 oranges.

Now, before the reader gains the impression that I spend an inordinate amount of time in fruit shops trying to decide how to deploy my fruit budget, it has to be emphasised that this is a model of how I behave. Given certain fixed prices for these goods, I perceive myself to be better off with this mix than if, say, the numbers above were in reverse order. Or again, assuming for simplicity that the prices of the two fruits are the same, then what emerges from my behaviour is that I would rather have this mix than, say, 99 avocados and 51 oranges, because the loss of the hundredth avocado is not compensated for by the gain of the fifty-first orange.

A point of importance in this is that the question of decision-making is 'at the margin'; that is, around the question of the hundredth avocado and the fiftieth orange. It is here that priorities are really sorted out. Thus, to prefer (or have higher priority for) avocados to oranges does not mean that I will always be buying avocados and no oranges. Nor indeed does it mean going on until the last one bought yields no benefit, because there is an opportunity cost in terms of foregone oranges. Thus, priorities are not absolute or 'lexicographic'; that is, we do not order our expenditure in such a way that we take care of our total want for our top priority, then move to our second priority, and so on. We adjust our consumption to try to make sure that we maximise benefit; we buy a little less of this and a little more of something else.

What if suddenly the price of avocados doubles? Now fewer avocados but more oranges will be bought because the opportunity cost of avocados (in terms of foregone oranges) has risen. Thus, the determination of the optimal use of my fruit budget is a function not only of my liking for oranges and avocados but also the relative costs of these products to me (in this case, money prices).

What the above discussion shows is that:

- Priorities neither are absolute nor follow a lexicographic ordering.
- Priorities are a function of both benefits and costs.
- The important area for decision-making is at the margin.
- The assessment of both costs and benefits is subjective.
- Different individuals may perceive costs and benefits (of the same things) differently.

In the context of health care, here are some examples of these economic messages:

- 'Priority for the elderly' does not mean devoting all expenditure or indeed all of any increased expenditure to the elderly, nor that we should fulfil the needs of the elderly *in toto* before considering other uses of resources.
- In deciding what and how much to do for the elderly, we should consider not only the benefits any action will provide but the costs (the opportunity costs) of foregoing benefits for the mentally ill, pregnant women, and so on.
- What priority setting means in practice is deciding whether we should spend an extra £1 million on the elderly, the mentally ill or pregnant women and then perhaps deciding whether we should spend another £1 million on the elderly, and so on.
- There are no scientifically objective measures of the benefits or costs of helping the elderly or any other client or patient group.
- Your perception of these costs and benefits may be quite different from mine.

2.2 Supply and demand: the market

Health care markets seem to operate rather differently from other markets. Nonetheless, it is important that readers have some understanding of how a basic market operates. It is not the intention to suggest that this model is appropriate to health care. Indeed, it will be argued later that markets for health care tend to fail for various reasons.

From the fact that resources are scarce and people's wants are seemingly insatiable emerges the important notions in economics of 'demand' and 'supply'. Demand is about how willing consumers are to pay for different goods and services. Supply is about the production side and how costs of factors of production and prices of the final product affect the amount of goods supplied. These ideas are relevant to health care, although not necessarily in the unbridled and sometimes rather naive form presented in this section. However, grasping the concepts presented here at least allows the reader to get hold of the basics of conventional economics; we can worry more about the application to health care later.

As consumers, we have various wants for goods and services that we desire (i.e. that would give us some positive satisfaction). Combining wants with limited income, we have the notion of (consumer) demand or willingness to pay.

Demand assumes that the best people to decide on the values to be attached to various goods and commodities are normally those who will benefit from them (i.e. the consumers). It assumes it is they who are the most knowledgeable and best placed to make the appropriate value judgements. It is from this notion that the important principle of 'consumer sovereignty' emerges, the idea that consumers should be sovereign on the demand side of the marketplace. (In Chapter 3, we will discuss the problems that arise when consumers are not very knowledgeable about the relevant commodities, as for example in health care.)

The demand curve for a good or service shows the relationship between its price and the quantity wished to be purchased (when income, tastes and the prices of all other goods and services are held constant). The nature of demand is such that it will normally be the case that the demand curve will slope downwards from left to right – indicating that the lower the price, the greater the quantity demanded (see Figure 2.1).

Lying behind demand is the concept of 'utility', which is economists' jargon for satisfaction. Economists assume that the greater the utility obtained from a visit to the cinema, the greater will be the price that anyone will be prepared to pay for it. The way that individuals deploy their incomes across the very wide range of goods and services available indicates some attempt to maximise utility.

If all goods were offered at the same price, it would be rational for the individual to consume those goods that had the greatest utility attached to them. However, this would not necessarily mean consuming one of each of such goods, because

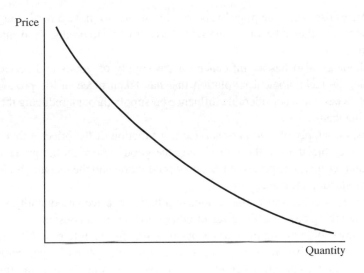

Figure 2.1 Downward-sloping demand curve

more utility might be obtained from the consumption of, say, two oranges and one apple than from one orange, one apple and one pear.

It is at this point that the concept of 'marginal utility' comes into play, in particular 'diminishing marginal utility'. Thus, if I consume two oranges a day, my utility will be greater than if I consume only one. But it is unlikely that I will obtain twice as much utility. Thus, if we say that marginal utility is the additional utility from consuming one extra unit of a good, then diminishing marginal utility means simply that, as more and more of a particular good is consumed, the utility obtained from each additional unit of consumption will tend to fall.

To maximise my utility, what I want to ensure is that the last pound spent on each good yields the same utility to me. If this is not the case and I get more utility from the last pound I spend on carrots than from the last pound spent on sprouts, then I can increase my overall utility by spending more on carrots and less on sprouts. It has to be emphasised that this is a theory. It is not intended to be a description of consumers' thinking when they go out shopping. It is the 'as if' principle; that is, consumers behave *as if* they were thinking along these lines.

While different objectives can be specified for producers of goods and services, economists frequently assume that producers attempt to maximise profits – the difference between what they receive from selling their goods (revenue) and what it costs the producer to make the goods (production costs). The higher prices are, all other things being equal, the more profit the supplier of the goods will make. The prices of other goods can affect the supply of a particular good. This is because, if other prices rise while the price of the good in which we have a particular interest remains steady, then it becomes relatively less attractive to producers to supply this particular good.

Technology also has an influence on the supply of goods and services. For example, the technological revolution that has taken place in the production of computers has had a considerable influence on supply through reducing the cost of producing them.

Thus, the supply of a good or service is a function of the price of that good or service, the objectives of those producing the good or service, the prices of other goods and services, the prices of factors of production and the technology involved in the production processes.

The supply curve shows the relationship between price and quantity supplied, when everything else (e.g. the price of other goods) is held constant.

But why should the supply curve slope upwards from left to right? It is simply a question of incentives for the producer. The higher the price of a particular good, the more resources the producer will be prepared to devote to producing that good. Therefore, if the price of apples rises, and nothing else changes, the producer of apples can increase their profits by putting more resources into the production of apples and fewer into, say, the production of pears. The producer might also convert some of their orchard from pear trees to apple trees if they believe that the new price is likely to be sustained.

Just as utility lies behind the concept of demand, so cost lies behind the concept of supply. A firm will supply goods of a particular type only if it can at least cover its costs. This is why there is a basic relationship between price and quantity supplied. The higher the price, the more costs are likely to be met and the greater the profits to be obtained. Supply and demand can now be brought together in the context of market prices, as in Table 2.1 for potatoes.

Table 2.1 Six situations in the market for potatoes

Situation	Price of potatoes per ton (£s)	Quantity demanded per month (tons)	Quantity supplied per month (tons)	Excess demand (+)/ excess supply (−) (tons)
i	100	500	180	+320
ii	150	400	240	+160
iii	200	320	320	0
iv	250	260	400	−140
v	300	220	500	−280
vi	350	200	620	−420

In situation (i) the price per ton of potatoes is £100. At this price the quantity demanded per month is 500 tons but the quantity supplied per month is only 180 tons. Thus, there is excess demand. Similarly, in situation (ii) there is an excess demand of 160 tons (400 tons–240 tons). In both situations there will be frustrated potential purchasers, at least some of whom will be prepared to bid up prices in an attempt to obtain more potatoes. Further, producers will be aware that they could raise their prices and still sell all their potatoes. There is thus pressure from both consumers and producers to raise the price of potatoes.

In situations (iv), (v) and (vi) there is excess supply. Producers will be faced with unsold potatoes unless they lower their prices, and consumers, becoming aware that the market is flooded with potatoes, will be less prepared to pay high prices for potatoes. There is thus pressure from both consumers and producers to reduce the price of potatoes.

When demand is greater than supply, there will be pressure to increase price; when supply is greater than demand, there will be pressure to reduce price. When there is neither excess demand nor excess supply (i.e. the market is in equilibrium), there will be no pressure to increase or decrease price. In Table 2.1 the equilibrium price is £200 per ton.

2.3 Economic evaluation

This section formulates a little more rigorously what has been said about evaluation and priority setting. As Samuelson's last sentence in his definition of economics indicates, economists are much concerned with the weighing-up of costs and benefits in health care and elsewhere. Certainly it would be wrong to suggest that health economics equals cost–benefit analysis (CBA) of health and health care. Yet of all the techniques of economic analysis available to the practitioner in the system, economic evaluation is perhaps the most relevant. The cost–benefit approach (or 'economic evaluation', as it is sometimes called) is already fairly well known in health care circles. This is not surprising. For can anyone deny the essential truths of CBA – that we should do only those things where benefits exceed costs, that the judgement as to what constitutes costs and benefits should be made on the broadest of social canvasses, and that the valuation of benefits and costs is normally best made by those who are advantaged and disadvantaged by their existence?

Despite these truths, it remains the case that the understanding of the principles of the cost–benefit approach remains poor in health care. The practice is rather infrequent and often of low quality. Here I want to spell out briefly what the principles are. Why there are problems in practice will become apparent as the book proceeds. The problems will be addressed explicitly in the final chapter, together with some suggestions on how they can be overcome.

The cost–benefit approach deals with two concepts of efficiency, and here we need a little jargon: 'technical efficiency' and 'allocative efficiency'. The former accepts a particular objective as given and is then concerned only with how to meet this objective at least cost. The technique used to address this question of 'how' is cost-effectiveness analysis (CEA).

Allocative efficiency is addressed by the technique of CBA, which considers how to maximise the benefit from available resources. In this case, objectives are not predetermined, and each objective has to fight with all others to be implemented. Thus, CBA deals with the question of 'whether'. In the form of what has been called 'marginal analysis' – with issues 'at the margin' of programmes – CBA also helps in considering the question of 'how much'. CBA is performed on a wide canvas. *All* costs and benefits arising as a result of implementing a particular project, no matter on whom they fall, are relevant. This is because in health care we are concerned with the welfare of society at large and not simply the health service. Thus, economists would argue that it is too narrow to consider increased community care purely in terms of the health effects on the clients and the costs to the health service since there are likely to be implications for other social services (e.g. local authority social work departments), for the clients in other than health effects (e.g. cost of living in the community), and for clients' relatives (e.g. a son or daughter doing some of the caring in the community). The viewpoint is thus a societal one.

With CEA it will normally be the case that the costs will be defined more narrowly, often purely in terms of those falling on the health service budget. In practice, however, a wider view of costs is often taken, similar to that adopted in CBA.

Since CBA attempts to help us to decide whether something should be done, there are two important principles on which it is founded:

- Do only those things where benefits exceed costs.
- Do not do those things where costs exceed benefits.

It follows that, since costs are often measured in money terms, to make them commensurate, economists also want to measure benefits in money terms. Clearly, CEA, which requires only some physical and not monetary measure of output or effectiveness, has the advantage over CBA of not getting into the difficult emotive realms of benefit valuation. But it is more restrictive in the questions it can address, particularly since in practice it has difficulty in coping with more than one output. (This is because once there is more than one output, assuming they do not always vary directly with each other, then relative weights have to be attached to these different outputs.)

In these circumstances another form of analysis comes into play – cost–utility analysis (CUA). This uses a multidimensional measure of health, usually called the quality adjusted life year (QALY), on the output side. This attempts to combine quantity of life with quality of life in a single index. Clearly, in so far as it can succeed in achieving this, there are great advantages over the single-dimensional output with which cost-effectiveness studies can deal. More detailed discussion of QALYs per se follows in Chapter 4.

CUA also allows, under certain restrictive assumptions, a way of approaching allocative efficiency, essentially, which programmes – the elderly, the mentally ill, etc. – should get priority for but avoiding the necessity of going as far as CBA and the problems in that form of analysis that arise from the need to value the outputs in money terms. Indeed, it is at least partly because of these advantages that CUA has become rather popular in the last few years.

But there are problems. Those related specifically to QALYs will be discussed in Chapter 4. Here, briefly, I will simply mention some of the problems of CUA even if QALYs are taken to be an acceptable measure of health.

CUA assumes that there are no other objectives to health care than health maximisation. Yet there may be other aspects that people care about, e.g. information, and that QALYs would not cover.

There are usually equity objectives in health care and it is far from clear that CUA handles these issues well. CUA tends to be restricted to health service resources on the cost side. Indeed, it can be argued that it has to be. This is because, if we are saying that the goal of health services is to maximise health, then clearly within the health service budget, if health can be bought more cheaply with programme A than programme B we should first invest in programme A. The opportunity cost is wholly in terms of health. But if we allow other costs to be included, such as those falling on patients, then the opportunity cost of, for example, patient time may be in all sorts of things and not just health.

To be clear on these points: CUA, assuming that QALYs measure health adequately, can be used to promote allocative efficiency provided that we are not concerned with equity; provided that the output of health services is purely health and nothing else; and provided that we are interested only in the efficiency with which health service resources are used and not the resources, such as those of patients, outside the health service. This is not to be overcritical of CUA but simply to put it into perspective in terms of some of the restrictions on its use. It should be noted, too, that these restrictions apply primarily to its use in the context of allocative efficiency.

In marginal analysis, the same basic rules apply as in CBA, except that they are now applied 'at the margin'. If no budget constraint exists, then a programme should be expanded or contracted to the point where marginal benefit equals marginal cost; if there is a budget constraint, then all programmes should operate at a level whereby the ratio of marginal benefit to marginal cost is the same for all. (This 'law' is the same as saying that the last pound spent on each programme should yield the same benefit and is the equivalent of the maximising utility point on page 7.)

When costs and benefits occur in time matters. For example, even in an inflationless world faced with paying, say, £220 for a television set now or being able to have the set but delaying the payment for one year, I would prefer the latter. I still get the benefit of the set from now but the cost to me is less because I can invest £200 *now* and with interest have £220 available in a year's time. In other words, the *present* value of the cost is £200, not £220.

Let's say that, if I had to pay £220 now, I would not buy the set; if £200 now, I would buy it. The fact that the present value of the cost is £200 and not £220 makes the difference between buying and not buying. In other words, I weigh up the present value of the stream of benefits (pleasure) I expect to get from the set against the present value of the costs, and if the former exceeds the latter, I buy; if not, I don't.

This process works equally well on the benefit side but, in a sense, in reverse. Benefits in the future are valued at less than benefits in the present. Perhaps we need to recognise that in addition to the investment argument (which is simply another facet of the concept of opportunity cost), as individuals we have a preference for 'good' things now rather than later (and the reverse with 'bad' things). This may be because of a simple time-preference (psychologically), but in addition there are the factors of uncertainty (e.g. we might die or our tastes might have changed in the future) and the idea of 'diminishing marginal utility of income'. This slightly awesome expression simply means that an extra £100 is likely to have a higher value if our current income is £500 than if it is £50,000. Assuming that our real incomes will increase through time, then this is another argument for 'discounting' the future.

This process of discounting is particularly important where the *timing* of costs and benefit is very different. For example, in preventive programmes (such as many screening services), there may be a gap of several years between when the major costs are incurred and when the benefits will arise. Because of the need to discount, this will have the effect of reducing the present value of the benefits much more than that of the costs. (It might be argued that this explains why antismoking campaigns for young people have tried to move away from emphasising the long-term benefits of mortality reduction to more short-term benefits, such as smokers not being as appealing to the opposite sex.)

Both costs and benefits are subjective concepts. It is frequently possible to assume that the costs of, say, nursing time are represented fairly accurately by the wages and overheads associated with the employment of nurses. Other costs may be very difficult or even impossible to value (e.g. the time spent by a son or daughter in looking after an ageing parent). However, even when values cannot be assigned, at least noting these intangible costs means that they are less likely to be lost sight of in any decision taken.

On the benefit side, there are problems in measuring and valuing health (an issue covered in greater detail in Chapters 4 and 5). But the essence of the value question here is that it cannot be avoided. Any decision to spend £1 million on saving a life means that the life is being valued at at least £1 million; a decision *not* to proceed implies a value of less than £1 million.

Related to the issue of how to value is that of who should do the valuing. Returning to my half-marathon training and my purchase of avocados, decisions about time and expenditure of resources devoted to them are probably best left to me. (Who knows better than I do the benefits of these activities to me and the opportunity costs involved for me?) This is known as 'consumer sovereignty', a concept dear to the hearts of many economists. But in health care, particularly in a public health service, is the 'consumer' best placed to decide on their consumption of health care? Certainly most of us may be prepared to accept on occasions that 'the doctor knows best'. Does this mean that doctors' sovereignty should apply in health care? Perhaps – but bear in mind that at least part of the reason why health care is generally not available in an unregulated marketplace is born of the view that we ought not to leave decision-making in this important area of life to doctors, patients or some combination of these parties. Should we then have politicians' sovereignty in health care?

Answers to these questions are central to the debate about the nature, organisation and financing of health care. Given that, they are clearly also important to the theme of this book. Consequently, these questions are addressed in more detail in later chapters.

2.4 Conclusion

Economics is about choice; it is about opportunity cost; it is about maximising the benefit to society from the resources available.

The goal is efficiency – getting the most we can out of the available labour, land and capital, often tempered by some concern with equity. The viewpoint is society's at large and not any single individual's or individual group's perspective. The ethic is that of the common good and, indeed, not settling for doing good but doing better, more fairly.

It is therefore unfortunate that economics has been dubbed the dismal science. More accurately, it is the joyful art since it attempts to maximise social benefit from the resources available subject to reasonable concerns with justice. It is thus the task of economists to spread a little happiness or, more accurately, to spread as much happiness as resources will permit – a laudable goal indeed. Fascinating, then, that in health care, where caring and humanitarian instincts pervade discussion and action, there is a reluctance to embrace this joyful art. Is economics getting it wrong? Is health care not about efficiency (i.e. about delivering the best/most health possible)? Are doctors not the caring people we all believe them to be? Or do they care about something else?

Of key significance to efficiency in any economic system is the knowledge required by the actors. Indeed, good information is the basis of the freedom that proponents of market economics suggest is one of its greatest virtues. Yet in health care there has to be concern about the extent and distribution of knowledge, and consequently the success in pursuing efficiency and in turn the nature and protection of freedom.

These issues are central to this book. We will return to them. In the meantime we need to investigate the nature of health and health care. It is to this that the next chapter is devoted.

Questions

1. In just a few words, how would you define economics?
2. What are the two *key* concepts of economics?
3. Do you have lexicographic preferences for oranges over avocados?
4. Does you preference for avocados change with price? Does your demand?
5. What does the mouthful 'diminishing marginal utility' mean?
6. What question(s) does cost–benefit analysis address?
7. Why do we discount the future?

Notes

1. P.A. Samuelson, *Economics* (McGraw-Hill: Tokyo, 1976), p 5.

three

The nature of the commodity health care

Perhaps what is most unique to health care is the knowledge on the part of both doctor and patient that the knowledge gap exists.

3.1 Introduction

One of the central issues in health care is that of deciding how to value health. Since resources are limited in all health services and the need for health care is dynamic and ever increasing, value judgements are required about priorities. What health service objectives should get higher weight? Should the acute services get more or fewer resources? Should the elderly get more or fewer resources? Who should have a transplanted kidney, and who should not? Should all mothers have their babies delivered in hospital (indeed, in a specialist maternity unit)?

This chapter begins a discussion on some of the issues involved in valuation of health – problems associated with health and health care per se, problems of ethics and measurement, problems of demand and consumer sovereignty, problems of measuring health and problems of actually placing values on health outputs such as lives saved. Aspects of these issues are debated further in Chapters 4–6.

Economists have been much intrigued in recent years by the nature of the 'commodity' health care, particularly in trying to explain why markets ('non-markets' may be a more appropriate description) for health care differ from those for most other goods. It can be frustrating (at least, for economists) to discover that textbook economics does not explain very well the market for health care in terms of conventional supply and demand analysis, as spelt out in the previous chapter. It may seem a little strange that anyone should want to consider health and health care alongside avocados, golf clubs and concerts, but this is the way in which economists tend to think. This chapter attempts to show that much of relevance to debates about health care policy can be gleaned by an examination of some of the rather peculiar attributes of health and health care. I will first consider health and then turn to health care.

3.2 Defining health

It is interesting and perhaps significant in terms of the difficulty of the task that we need to begin by asking what health is. Yet we must because it is a concept that is difficult to define and that is subject to many different interpretations, some of which, but only some, are relevant to our discussion.

The World Health Organization defines health as 'a state of complete physical, mental and social well-being, and not merely the absence of disease or infirmity'.[1] Such a definition, while one with which it is only too easy to agree, is difficult to operate with in practice if we are to attempt to consider the nature of health and later the measurement and valuation of health.

To most medical doctors, fascinatingly, the question of defining health and ill-health is of little, if any, relevance to them. That is perhaps understandable. Doctors deal with death and disease on a daily basis so the idea of taking time to define health or even ill health must seem not only abstract to many doctors but also somewhat pointless.

Yet it matters. This is especially true when we think of health policy at some aggregate level. After all, if health cannot be defined, or maybe more relevantly if health cannot be measured, then what? What do we do with respect to performance indicators for the health system? Is health overall going up or down? Are we getting healthier as a nation?

There can be major differences in how health is viewed, and the weight attached to these differing views in different contexts is important. The issue of the individual doctor's perception and the broader community perspective is first raised here. It is an issue that will plague us all the way through this book, just as it plagues all debates about health care policy. It is central to the issue of medical ethics and its conflict with rational resource allocation. Yet it is an issue that the medical profession individually and collectively tends to ignore or seeks to avoid.

Health can be viewed in several different ways. For example, Twaddle suggests that from a biological standpoint, 'perfect health' might be seen as 'a state in which every cell of the body is functioning at optimum capacity and in perfect harmony with each other cell'.[2] Again from a social standpoint, 'perfect health may be a state in which an individual's capacities for taste and role performance are optimised'.

The concepts of health and sickness can be very different depending upon the definition used and particularly the standpoint adopted. Thus, according to Twaddle, 'there is a wide consensus among medical people that illness is any state that has been diagnosed as such by a competent professional ... Alternatively, there is a view that whoever feels ill should be regarded as sick.' These different definitions and the different standpoints from which they emerge are of much importance in considering the nature of health and later health care as a commodity.

3.3 Health and health care

We can circumvent some of the problems here by suggesting that the real interest of this book and what is central to our debate is the demand and supply of health care rather than health per se. But we need to be careful lest the impression be given that the two can be seen as wholly separate.

First, there seems little value in health per se. Rather, its value stems from its possession, allowing us to act out more fulfilling lives in terms of work and play than we might do otherwise. This immediately leads to various complications in that to be interested in the concept of health means to be interested in all aspects of life from which individuals derive satisfaction, since in extreme ill health all of these may be snuffed out. Add in the fact that ill health itself comes in many guises – pain, physical disability, mental impairment, and so on, each with differing degrees of severity – and the problems grow, becoming infinitely greater once we accept that a nominally equal state of ill health may have very different implications for different individuals. The loss of a leg or an arm would clearly create considerably greater problems for a professional footballer or a classical pianist, respectively, than for a health economist. Thus, the demand for health is largely a derived demand, derived from the value we place on being fit and well to lead fulfilling lives.

Second, while health (however defined) is supplied by health care systems, it is also supplied through many other agencies. Indeed, it might be argued that the main supplier of health for any individual is the individual him or herself through sensible diet, exercise, and so on. Health is also supplied through prevention of road accidents, clean air regulations, occupational health and safety regulations, and building regulations. We ought not to lose sight of this fact.

Third, there is a definite if often ill-specified relationship between health and health care. While we can promote our own health in many ways, for most of us it is difficult to envisage any other reason for approaching the health care system than for reasons of health promotion. There is a sense in which any demand we have for health care is derived from our demand for health; that is, we are prepared to lie in a hospital bed not because we enjoy it per se but because we hope that by doing so we will attain a higher level of health. The demand for health care is thus also a derived demand, derived from our demand for health in so far as the health care system can, as we see it, promote that health.

Related to these broad issues of the demand for health and the demand for health care, one economist, Grossman, in what has become a classic article, has suggested that the way that we view health ought to be as a durable capital asset that is a fundamental commodity underlying many others.[3] This approach is based on the notion that health is produced by households, each household having a demand for health that may or may not on occasion become a demand for health care.

In this way, households have demands for many goods that may not necessarily or always be desired solely for their own sake. For example, food, housing and physical exercise are demanded at least in part for their health-producing attributes. This idea of seeing the demand (willingness to pay) for goods as the demand for the different attributes of the good can be useful in a number of instances. Thus, while many smokers do realise that smoking is bad for their health (there is some negative utility in the sense that they would be willing to pay to *remove* this attribute), this is more than compensated for by the positive utility from the other attributes of smoking. (If we make cigarettes 'safer', almost certainly the number of cigarettes smoked will increase, not because smokers are perverse but simply because the demand for a safe product is likely to be greater than the demand for a risky one. This may be a partial explanation for what happened when filter cigarettes came on the market.)

Thus, in this view the focus is on the household, with the formal health care sector coming into play only when the household demands it as part of its demand for health. This is a potentially useful way of considering health and points perhaps to the need for the formal health care services to do more to promote awareness of the health-producing activities that go on outside the health care sector. (More tangibly, it might be argued that what the job of health educationalists or prevention officers in health care should be is to mobilise resources for health from *outside* the formal health care sector.) There are dangers in the approach, however. Certainly let's try to persuade people to eat apples if it is healthy to do so, but it is important to appreciate at the same time that, if we suddenly discover new evidence to suggest that apples are carcinogenic, we are likely to affect not just the demand for the health attributes of apples but of many other goods as well. This is a form of 'externality', the importance of which I suspect is much underestimated. Am I alone in discounting statements about what is good or bad for me in my diet because there has been so much misinformation issued in recent years by the medical profession and other 'experts' about possible harm from different foodstuffs, additives, and so on? Rightly or wrongly, I still eat butter, and if I'm told tomorrow that Guinness is not good for me, I will tend to discount the information because of all the conflicting information I have received previously on butter and margarine – and also because I like Guinness for its other characteristics as well.

But perhaps more serious is the fact that such a model tends to assume a high degree of rationality on the part of the consumer and a well-informed household. Whether such assumptions are justified must be debatable. However, these are not reasons for rejecting the notion of the household's 'health durable asset', particularly in the context of non-health-care health-producing activities, where in any case, whether we like it or not, the consumer will tend to be sovereign.

In practice, many of the non-health-care health commodities are prevention goods. Thus, while most forms of cure are vested in the formal health care system, the majority of prevention consumption is elsewhere. Some of it is organised by recognised agencies – road safety, clean air, river pollution control, and so on. Other aspects are the subject of legislation, normally, interestingly, to constrain 'bad' consumption (e.g. it is illegal to use certain drugs, or to drink more than a certain amount of alcohol and then drive a motor vehicle; cigarettes and alcohol are taxed to reduce the quantity demanded) rather than to promote 'good' consumption (e.g. why don't we have a subsidy or negative tax on jogging shoes, wholemeal bread and polyunsaturated fats?). Again, in other instances the market and the consumer are left to get on with it.

In examining non-health-care health-promoting activities, it becomes apparent that many commodities have some either health-promoting ('preventive') attributes or health-diminishing ('hazardous') attributes. This is clear with, for example, smoke-detecting devices. But for some brands of margarine, not only do they taste nice on bread and toast; they also have the characteristic of being more health-promoting than their close substitute butter. Swimming is not only enjoyable as a sport; it also promotes fitness (it also has the health-diminishing characteristic of there being some risk of drowning associated with it).

Consequently, the demand for health can be very complex. As exhibited in health care, it is subject to considerable problems of lack of knowledge and lack of rationality on the part of the consumer. Outside of health care the demand is exhibited as that for various health-promoting and health-diminishing facets of all sorts of different types of commodities. For the former, we tend in society to organise the health care system in such a way as to assist and moderate consumer demand so that individuals are more likely to get it 'right' than if left to their own devices. In the equally complex world of non-health-care health-promoting/health-diminishing consumption, except where the effects are both clearly discernible and potentially disastrous (and of course that word can be subjected to all sorts of different interpretations), consumers are much freer to make their own mistakes. There would seem to be an inconsistency here.

In addition to the externality of misinformation on risk, two other forms of externality exist concerning health. There is the consideration that, if you have an infectious disease, then your state of health may directly affect mine. This is an issue of much less importance today, at least in developed countries, than it has been in the past. (But it is not absent. When one of my colleagues has a cold, my suggestion that they take the day off and return to bed is born of concern for my being infected as well as for their poor health.) AIDS – and most recently SARS – has clearly important externalities. Here, also, we have the second externality. To a greater extent than in other aspects or characteristics of our fellow beings, we do appear to be concerned for the health of others. This 'humanitarian spill-over' does seem to be an important form of externality that, while not unique to health (we can be concerned for the poor, for example), is more pervasive (we care about the rich as well as the poor being ill) and stronger (we are probably more likely to give, at the margin, to charities concerned with alleviating ill health than those aimed at alleviating poverty). It is interesting to note that, even with a public health service, there are still many people who donate funds and give their time to buy dialysis machines, scanners, TV sets for hospitals, and so on. Indeed, this humanitarian spill-over has been suggested as one of the fundamental reasons for the UK National Health Service being established. Before leaving health I would also point to what I think is an increasingly important aspect of discussions in this area. This is the tendency to consider that health in itself is 'a good thing'. Health is clearly value-laden (something we will consider in detail in the next chapter). But what this means is that individuals may well value it differently and make different trade-offs between different aspects of health. Some people, for example, may prefer a short and handicap-free life, while others would opt for a longer life but with a handicap.

These considerations are very much concerned with values. And this needs to be recognised. At the same time there is a need to accept that in 'advocating' health or healthy lifestyles there may be some disadvantages to this in terms of increasing individuals' anxiety levels. For example, cholesterol-lowering policies may result in reduced heart disease but at the same time they may increase the level of anxiety in the population as a result of telling people what their cholesterol levels are.

3.4 Health care

The nature of the commodity health care has been examined by a number of economists. In discussing this, I wish to acknowledge my debt to, in particular, the early work by Arrow,[4] Culyer[5] and Williams.[6]

Economics, as discussed in the context of demand in Chapter 2, normally starts from the point of view of consumer sovereignty; that is, that the individual is the best judge of his or her own interests. Then there may be some relaxation of these assumptions. For example, my consumption of alcohol can have implications for others ('externalities') in that I may indulge in antisocial activities such as drunken driving. The government may then intervene and pass laws to penalise me if I drink and drive, to protect not so much myself as others. Thus, government may interfere in different ways to influence consumption decisions by individuals.

But a second problem of this type is rather important in the context of health care. There may be, as Arrow suggests and as is discussed in the context of medical ethics in Chapter 7, 'a discrepancy, real or fancied, between the decisions an individual would reach on his own and those that he should reach to increase his own welfare. In short, he may be ill informed about what is good for him.'[7] As Arrow indicated, this is the classic paternalistic argument.

The basic point with regard to health care is that there is a major asymmetry in information between the doctor and the patient. The results of this are that, first, the patient's ability to make their own decisions is impaired and, second, the patient becomes very much dependent on the doctor to make decisions on their behalf. What is crucial is that the patient has little check on the doctor, when the doctor is determining the patient's 'need' (of which more in Chapter 6).

Part of the explanation for this, but largely a separate issue, is the fact that the demand for health care is both irregular and unpredictable. Add to this the fact that illness is not only risky (e.g. with some probability of death) but also financially expensive. While some of these items of irregularity, unpredictability and high financial cost may be observed in markets for other goods, it is difficult to think of any other where they are all present.

There is also considerable uncertainty regarding the quality of the product. Not only is it difficult for the doctor to judge on many occasions the probability of a particular outcome (and obviously even more difficult for the patient), but there is also the added difficulty for the patient of not being able to judge whether the doctor has done a good job. This is very different from the market for avocados, where the quality of the product is as well known to the regular consumer as it is to the producer.

The issue of the behaviour expected by the patient of the doctor is also an important consideration and arises in a sense because of all the points already made, particularly the question of differential information. However, the key factor here is not the differential information per se but rather the knowledge of both parties – doctor and patient – that the differential exists.

Arrow[7] lists four ways in which the expected behaviour of the doctor is different from that expected of the typical businessperson:

- Advertising and overt competition are virtually eliminated among physicians.
- Advice given by the physician as to further treatment by himself or others is supposed to be completely divorced from self-interest.
- It is claimed that treatment is dictated by the objective needs of the case and not limited by financial considerations.
- The physician is relied on as an expert in certifying to the existence of illness and injuries for various legal and other purposes. It is socially expected that the physician's concern for the correct conveying of information will, when appropriate, outweigh their decision to please their customers.

It is interesting to note that while the nature, organisation and financing of health care systems differ in many respects between countries, as far as I can judge, although Arrow was writing specifically about the US health care system, all of his points appear valid to other health care systems as well. Further, we may note that, given these circumstances, it is hardly surprising that even in the USA the profit motive in health care is comparatively weak (with many more not-for-profit than for-profit hospitals).

Turning more directly to the supply side, there are a number of features of interest in health care markets in comparison with normal competitive markets. Clearly, entry to the medical profession (as is true of many others) is restricted. This results in raising both the quality and the cost of medical care.

A related phenomenon on the supply side is that restriction of entry results in a restriction in the *range* of quality. In many markets, it is possible to find varying quality (and normally, therefore, price) for particular types of commodities. But this is much less marked in medicine. Clearly, however, there have been some attempts to substitute less highly trained (and hence less costly) personnel for some tasks previously undertaken by medical staff.

In normal markets, prices play an important role. In health care, their influence is usually muted, although in some instances it can be enhanced. For example, the greengrocer cannot discriminate in prices between rich and poor, but under at least some health care systems such price discrimination by income is both possible and practised. Pricing policy also comes into play in terms of doctor remuneration, where in different countries, and sometimes even in the same country, doctors can be paid salaries, on a per capita basis or on a fee-for-service basis.

But perhaps the most significant aspect of all on pricing policies in health care in all countries is that price competition, which is normally seen as a virtue in other markets, is considered a vice. It is deemed unethical for the medical profession to indulge in price competition.

The existence in many countries of some form of health insurance also affects the 'market' for health care. Once the premium is paid, prices at the point of consumption are either zero or heavily subsidised, with the inevitable consequences of higher quantities of health care demanded than would otherwise be the case.

Given these problems on both the demand side and the supply side for the commodity of health care, it is not surprising that markets for health care tend to be rather different from markets for other commodities. Indeed, the way that health care is supplied varies markedly from country to country, even within the industrialised West, stretching on the one hand from the UK *National* Health Service to the more market-oriented system of the USA, from salaried systems for the medical profession to fee-per-item of service, from zero money prices at the point of consumption to substantial co-payment by consumers, and so on.

There is no general agreement on how best to deliver health care. Indeed, it is striking that while medical technology knows no boundaries, in the sense that it is genuinely international in its availability and consumption, that is less true of the technology of health care delivery. While there has been a shift in this respect in the last 20 years, we are much more ignorant about other countries' systems of health care than we are about their medical technology. Even where we have some knowledge, we struggle to form judgements about the relative value of different systems.

This is getting better. More countries are reforming or considering reforming their health care systems. As a result, there is a growing recognition that we can learn from how other countries organise their health care.

3.5 Conclusion

A number of points emerge from this chapter; for example, that the nature of health care will vary depending on the way in which health care is organised and financed. This may in turn be a function of ideological and cultural variations between countries. The method of remuneration of the medical profession will also have major implications for the demand and supply of health care.

It is clear, however, that while no single feature or characteristic of health care is unique to health care, there are few if any goods that have all the characteristics of uncertainty, irrationality, unpredictability, large monopoly elements, paternalism and important externalities. To those who doubt that health care is different, the question must be posed of why it is that it gets *treated* differently from lawnmowers, transport, education, books, and so on.

Indeed, it is the combination of all these factors that makes health care unique as a commodity. Within these factors, perhaps the most important is the knowledge gap between patient and doctor and, perhaps even more significantly, what might be termed the 'knowledge squared gap' – the knowledge by both parties that the knowledge gap exists. As is discussed in Chapter 7, it is this that largely explains the existence of medical ethics, and it is this that explains almost wholly the importance of medical ethics. Not all, however, would necessarily agree that economics can be of much assistance in analysing health care (see, for example, Kernick[8]).

Another important issue which emerges from this chapter is the question of how we are to grapple with the problems of measuring and valuing health. This we discuss in the next three chapters.

Questions

1. Is the value of the loss of a leg constant?
2. The demand for health care is derived from what?

3. As compared with other commodities, how sits the demand for health care?
4. What is an 'externality'? Give a couple of examples.
5. What is the 'knowledge squared gap'?
6. Can 'quality' in health care be judged? Easily? By whom?
7. Can patients define their own need?

Notes

1. World Health Organization, *Constitution* (WHO: New York, p 1.).
2. A.C. Twaddle, 'The concept of health status', *Social Science and Medicine*, 8 (1974), p 31.
3. M. Grossman, 'On the concept of health capital and the demand for health', *Journal of Political Economy*, 80 (1972), pp 223–255.
4. K.J. Arrow, 'Uncertainty and the welfare economics of medical care', *American Economic Review*, 53 (1963), pp 941–973.
5. A.J. Culyer, 'The nature of the commodity health care and its efficient allocation', *Oxford Economic Papers*, 23 (1971), pp 189–211.
6. A. Williams, 'Medicine, ethics and the NHS: a clash of cultures?' *Health Economics*, 7 (1998), pp 565–568.
7. Arrow, op.cit.
8. D.P. Kernick, 'A new journal on the block: unorthodox, troublesome and dangerous, or just more of the same', *Applied Health Economics and Health Policy*, 1 (2002), pp 3–5.

four

Health status and other outcome measurement

A nail factory met its target of 100 tons of nails by fabricating nails of 1 kilo each. The planners saw their error and instructed the factory to maximize the number of nails. The nails were too small to be of use.

H. Oxley, 'Rainbows and pots of gold: the search for public sector efficiency', Public Sector Workshop: Helsinki (1991)

4.1 Introduction

Health status measurement and valuation are two of the most important and most difficult aspects of health care evaluation generally and of health economics in particular. Essentially, measurement is difficult for three reasons: (1) health is a value-laden concept; (2) health is multidimensional; and (3) it is normally not enough to be able to measure health ordinally – we need cardinal measurement.

Ordinality and cardinality (on both an interval and a ratio scale) are discussed in this chapter before considering the measurement of health status. First, there is emphasis on the need for different judgements – both technical and value judgements – by different 'actors' in the health care system. The link (and sometimes confusion) between ordinality and cardinality is highlighted and the way that an index can be devised is examined.

Second, the questions of QALYs and their measurement are set out at some length. These represent a particular form of health status measurement that have gained some popularity (and notoriety) in recent years.

Consideration is then given to the idea that there may be arguments in the patients' and the citizens' health care utility functions other than health.

4.2 Issues in measuring health

One of the main problems in any health care evaluation is that of measuring health or health status and changes therein. The problem is not peculiar to economic evaluation, and many people from different disciplines have turned their minds to the issue. Different types of approach have been adopted and different types of health indicator devised. Before considering an example, some general comments are worth making about health status measurement.

There are potentially many uses to which health indicators can be put. For example:

- To compare the health status of the populations in different countries and relative changes through time.
- To compare the relative health status of the population in different regions of a country; for example, in order to form judgements about the allocation of health service expenditure to different regions.
- To measure the effects of different forms of clinical practice.

Different types of indicator will be relevant depending on the use envisaged. This in turn raises two important aspects of health status measurement: first, the fact that it is value-laden and, second, the related issue of the dimensions to be adopted in measuring health in specific contexts.

This issue of being value-laden is of importance regarding the choice of dimensions since that choice should be made on the basis of ensuring that what is measured allows one to see the extent to which the objective of the policy is being pursued. For example, if in the care of the elderly health status is measured in terms of life expectancy alone, this implies that health policy in the care of the elderly is concerned solely with keeping the elderly alive. (Clinicians are perhaps the biggest sinners in this respect. In cancer-control programmes, for example, despite various recent efforts to improve the position, it remains too often the case that the measures of health status they use are restricted to mortality.) If, however, a prior statement is made that health policy in caring for the elderly has the objective of assisting the elderly to function as well as possible in terms of social intercourse, looking after their own personal care, and so on, then measurements of health status might then be couched in terms of ability to go outdoors (alone, with aid, not at all), ability with personal care (able to wash alone, able to wash with aid, unable to wash), and so on. There are also different methods of indicating states of health. These fall broadly into two categories: ordinal and cardinal. An ordinal ranking system means simply that certain states of health are deemed to be better than others and, consequently, some are deemed to be worse than others. Thus, a health status index for the elderly would rank 'able to get out and about without an aid' as a higher (better, less severe) status than 'able to get out and about, but only with an aid', and 'able to get out and about, but only with an aid' as a higher (better, less severe) status than 'not able to get out and about at all'. If we ascribe numbers to these health statuses, with a high number denoting a good health status and a low number denoting a poor health status (it could be the other way about if we wanted), then we might have the following ordinal ranking:

1 = not able to get out and about
2 = able to get out and about, but only with an aid
3 = able to get out and about without an aid

Then 1 is worse than 2, 2 is worse than 3, and 1 is worse than 3. Notice that such an ordinal ranking says nothing about how much worse 1 is than 2 or how much better 3 is than 2.

While such an ordinal scale can be a useful starting point, ideally in most instances we would want to operate with cardinal scales so that we have some measure of the *difference* between points on the scale.

Essentially, there are two types of cardinal scales: interval scales and ratio scales. On an interval scale, the numbers ascribed to health statuses not only indicate ordinal ranking but also show that the interval between the numbers is the same. If the example of the scale for the elderly above was an interval scale, then we could say that to improve someone's health status from 1 to 2 would be as good as improving someone's health status from 2 to 3. We could not, however, say on an interval scale that it was three times better to have health status 3 than to have health status 1. To help grasp this, note that temperature is measured on an interval scale: thus, a change in temperature from 50 °C to 60 °C is equal to a change from 70 °C to 80 °C, i.e. both involve an increase of 10 °C. However, it is not legitimate to argue that 80 °C is 'twice as hot' as 40 °C or that 100 °C is '100 times as hot' as 1 °C. This is clear if we switch to Fahrenheit: the former is a change from 176 °F to 104 °F, the latter from 212 °F to 33.8 °F. The reason why interval scales do not permit this '*x* times' comparison is simply because the zero is fixed arbitrarily and has no meaning in itself. On a ratio scale, not only are the intervals between the numbers the same but we can also say that a health status of 10 is twice as good as a health status of 5 and five times as good as a health status of 2. (Distance is measured on a ratio scale: thus, ten metres is twice as long as five metres and five times as long as two metres.)

Different methods can be devised for arriving at different scales of health status. Essentially, however, in deciding whether a particular health status is better or worse than another (i.e. ordinal ranking), this involves a value judgement (which might, given the practical problems involved, have to be determined by a doctor, regardless of whether in principle this was thought to be the best source of values). Deciding how much better or worse (i.e. introducing cardinality) clearly involves another value judgement, and one that is much less likely to be the prerogative of the medical profession and that is more of a social judgement.

Let us consider an example. Someone with a cold has a lower/poorer health status than someone without a cold. Someone with pneumonia has lower health status than someone without either pneumonia or a cold or someone with a cold. These statements involve both value and technical judgements.

Now, let us say that it is possible to cure a cold at a cost of £50 and to cure pneumonia at a cost of £1000 (the cost difference being 20 times). If only £1000 is available, should we treat 20 colds or one case of pneumonia? If we value the change in health status from 'pneumonia' to 'no pneumonia' more than 20 times as highly as the change in health status from 'cold' to 'no cold', then we would treat the pneumonia case; if not, we would treat the colds. But deciding whether it is 20 times as bad to have pneumonia as having a cold is a value judgement.

The technical characteristics of a good health status index are as follows:

- Reliability and reproducibility i.e. reproducible by different people.
- Valid, i.e. it measures what it is supposed to measure.
- Able to be related to some of the variables over which the researcher or practitioner or administrator has some control.

4.3 Quality adjusted life years

There are many measures of health status. One way of trying to grapple in practice with health status measurement is through the use of QALYs. Seen from a health economics standpoint, QALYs represent one of the most controversial developments in health care evaluation in recent years. They have provoked much debate. Here I do not want to further the debate but rather to try to set out clearly what QALYs are about.

First, what are QALYs? They are a form of health status measurement that attempts to place mortality and morbidity on the same measuring rod. What is their function? In essence, QALYs have two main functions (although it is possible to extend this to many others, which have, in my view, lesser importance). First, they can allow more informed and rational judgements to be made about the effectiveness of one form of treatment for a particular problem as compared with another treatment for that same problem. Clearly, in economic terms, to be able to do so allows judgements to be made about technical efficiency. Is conventional surgery more efficient than laparoscopic cholecystectomy? Further, there are clear advantages in using this form of economic evaluation, cost–utility analysis (CUA), as compared with cost-effectiveness analysis (CEA), because CUA allows more than one type of health outcome to be included, whereas CEA is restricted to a unidimensional measure of outcome.

Table 4.1 QALY league table

Intervention	Present value of extra cost per QALY gained (£)
GP advice to stop smoking	170
Pacemaker implantation for heart block	700
Hip replacement	750
GP control of total serum cholesterol	1700
Kidney transplantation (cadaver)	3000
Breast cancer screening	3500
Heart transplantation	5000
Hospital haemodialysis	14 000

Source: Adapted from M.F. Drummond, 'Output measurement for resource allocation decisions in health care' in *Providing Health Care: The Economics of Alternative Systems of Finance and Delivery*, eds A. McGuire, P. Fenn and K. Mayhew (Oxford University Press: Oxford, 1991).

But more controversially, QALYs can be used in helping to judge relative priorities across different programmes in health care. Different types of treatment for different problems can be compared on the basis of 'marginal costs per QALY gained' and the increases in programmes with the 'cheapest' QALYs given highest priority. (This is on the basis that, with a fixed budget for health care, the goal is to maximise the number of QALYs within that budget, which in turn means buying the cheapest ones first. This is questioned later.)

It is for this purpose that the 'QALY league tables' (Table 4.1) have been devised. (For more discussion, see Chapter 9.) As explained, a few words of caution with regard to these tables are appropriate.

A final comment on QALYs per se is that they assume that what we want to measure is the value or utility associated with health state X, and then the utility of health state Y, and that the change in utility is given by the difference between these. In other words, the assessment of a health state is independent of the state of health one is in when one makes the assessment. (I may feel very different about being in a wheelchair depending on whether, when I make the judgement, I am reasonably fit and well – as of now – or I am already in the wheelchair.)

Yet I begin to fall into the trap of seeming to be very critical of QALYs. The reader should note two things here. First, the intention in setting out these opinions is not to knock QALYs down. Rather, it is to try to ensure that expectations with respect to them are realistic. Second, most of the reservations about QALYs relate to the question of QALY league tables and thus the use of QALYs with respect to allocative efficiency issues. Comparing different treatments for the same health problem is where the QALY can be supported almost unreservedly. And that is no mean recommendation, given that even today so many clinical evaluations are still performed using very inadequate measures of output. It is at the 'across programme' level that more problems are created. Not that that means we should drop QALYs at this level – just be aware of their limitations in this context. (For a debate on this issue, see, for example, Dowie,[1] Guyatt,[2] Feeny[3] and Brazier and Fitzpatrick.[4])

Now, even if the ordering seems a little odd, I want to turn to the measurement of QALYs. I have been quite deliberate in setting the ordering thus, because I have found so often that the measurement issues get in the way of the issues of principle with QALYs. If the reader becomes obsessed with the measurement issues, they may fail to appreciate the beauty (relatively, at least) of the principles incorporated in QALYs.

The history of QALYs is relatively long, but the key names associated with them are Torrance[5] in Canada and Williams[6] in the UK. In attempting to measure QALYs, what is being attempted is to devise some unidimensional scale that will allow both mortality and various forms and severity of morbidity to be placed on this single scale and in such a way that it is possible to compare health states with one another. This is to be done in the sense of saying not just that health state X is better than health state Y (i.e. ordinally) but also how much better (i.e. cardinally). What we want to be able to do is to add together health outputs and to compare the outputs in terms of costs per QALY from different ways of producing QALYs.

Here I want to set out, following Torrance, the three main ways of attempting to devise QALYs. These are the 'visual analogue scale' or the 'rating scale', the 'time trade-off' method, and the 'standard gamble'.

The first of these involves simply setting out a line on a page (or in some versions a thermometer) usually with one end equal to 0, equated with death, and the other end set at 1, equated with some best state of health. (For some people, there are states that are worse than death; for example, for Scots, living in England might be one.) The idea, then, is to get those asked to form judgements about other intermediate states of health to say where on the line these would lie. If, for example, losing the use of both legs is seen as being at 0.75, then this means that the respondent believes that the loss of the use of their legs reduces their health status vis à vis good health by one-quarter.

The time trade-off method is largely self-explanatory. It involves asking respondents to establish equivalents in terms of, for example, 20 years of life with the loss of the use of both legs followed immediately by death and X years of life with perfect health followed by immediate death. If the respondent then sets X equal to 15, the valuation of the health state 'loss of use of both legs' where 1 is perfect health is 0.75 (as in the example above using the rating scale).

The third approach, the standard gamble, is slightly more complex and involves facing the respondent with a pair of choices. One choice is remaining in their current (less than perfect) health state; the other involves some probability (p) of being immediately restored to perfect health and some probability (1 – p) of dying immediately. The respondent is asked to vary p until they are indifferent between the choices. If, for a current health state of the loss of use of both legs, the individual sets p equal to 0.75, then 0.75 is the valuation of this health state (when again death is 0 and perfect health is 1).

Which of these methods is to be preferred is the subject of considerable controversy. Clearly, if they all produced the same results, then the choice would not matter. Unfortunately, it appears that the measurements that emerge from the methods are not independent of the measuring method.

Additionally, there remains the question of who to ask. This takes us into the debate on 'whose values', which is picked up in the next chapter.

There has been a lot of debate in recent years about health status measurement, especially with respect to QALYs. Much of it seems to have been about two issues. First, there is the view that health status cannot be measured; second, even if it can be measured, QALYs are rather inadequate for doing so. What may be important to bear in mind here is that clinicians and policy-makers are implicitly making judgements about health status weights and measures daily. (It is simply not possible, for example, to draw up a contract for health services without implicitly at least measuring the expected health gains from contracting for one set of services as compared with another. Or at least one would hope that some idea of health status gains underlies any such contracting process!) Further, it is unlikely that there is anyone who would consider that the science or art of health status measurement has been perfected or that QALYs are the final word. There is a long way to go before we can be really confident that we are getting acceptable measures of what we want from QALYs. What is abundantly clear, however, is that what is currently done in health services by way of output measurement is really pretty dreadful and that, for many, QALYs represent a step in the right direction.

What has to be remembered constantly in all of this is that it really is very difficult to measure health well.

Am I being too defensive about QALYs? I think not. I have been rather critical of some of the work here myself and indeed have been taken to task by some of my health economist colleagues for this. But my criticisms are not intended to be anti-QALYs. They are aimed at trying to see whether we can get health care outcomes measured even better than current QALYs do and at pushing away the view that health economics is only about QALYs. My criticisms are also an attempt to make sure that we walk with QALYs rather than run too fast and face too much hostility, especially from the clinicians, in getting them used. There are problems and discussing them cannot do any harm – provided they are seen against the background of the need to improve on the way that health care outcomes are currently measured.

4.4 Other outcomes

Much of the literature on outcomes in health care is concerned solely with health, on the grounds either that that is the only outcome of the health care system or that health is the only one that is deemed relevant when examining health care policies from the standpoint of economic evaluation. In what follows, other possible arguments that may arise in patients' and citizens' utility functions are considered; in other words, what other health care features or characteristics may affect individuals' utilities?

Equity of access

QALYs as measures of health may not be enough, in so far as they do not consider equity, especially in the Margolis context of allowing a concern for 'doing our fair share'.[7] The Margolis model (see Chapter 10 for more detail) assumes that each individual has two utility functions, one concerned with a 'standard' neoclassical 'goods' utility function, the other with the utility derived from what Margolis calls 'participation utility'. Margolis assumes that individuals are prepared to contribute to 'group utility' (where each individual is a member of the group and as likely to obtain utility from the use of group resources as any other member of the group). They derive utility from the act of participating.

Here is a means of incorporating equity in health care within the individual's utility function. Individuals get utility from providing services that are then available to all. (All have access to them.) This utility arises from the act of provision – doing our fair share – rather than from the utility that the individuals in the group obtain from their use of these resources. This is particularly relevant when equity is so often defined in terms of access rather than of health care use or of health. The utility arises from the participation in the providing rather than in the use or in the health gains arising from such use. In more normal terminology, it arises through individuals contributing so that everyone has equal access to health care services.

One of the operational disadvantages of moving the equity target away from health per se is that it means that there is an argument in the utility function that concerns not health but access to health care.

It is not my intention to be normative here by implying that people ought to get utility from participation, or ought to get utility through improved equality of access. The point is rather to suggest that there may be an argument present in individuals' utility functions that goes beyond health. This would be seen in terms of contributing to the provision of health care to allow more equal access.

Information

In the context of the evaluation of a prenatal diagnostic test for autosomal polycystic kidney disease (APKD), I attempted, with Mette Lange, to show – and indeed would suggest that we have shown – that the individuals at risk whom we surveyed indicated a willingness to pay (quite substantial amounts) for information per se.[8]

Most at-risk individuals were willing to pay to have a test during pregnancy to show whether the affected gene was present in the fetus. For at-risk individuals, there is a 50 per cent chance that a fetus will be affected. If such an affected gene is present, this will mean that the individual will suffer from polycystic kidney disease. This will normally be symptomless until the age of about 40 or 50. Thereafter, it is likely to lead to end-stage renal disease, requiring either a kidney transplant or renal dialysis. Before the onset of end-stage renal disease, there is little that can be done to treat or slow the progression of the disease. Overall, therefore, the disease is very different from, say, Down's syndrome, and essentially it means a shortening of life expectation by perhaps ten years with relatively few morbidity effects.

Interestingly in the context of the utility of information, approximately half of the (admittedly small) sample were prepared to pay for the test without proceeding to choose to abort if the fetus was shown to be affected. Certainly it could be that this information was seen as relevant to the management of the birth and the impact on the woman of the discovery of the problem after birth. However, while this might seem a rational explanation if we were dealing with Down's syndrome, given the nature of APKD this seems unlikely. We argue that this represents utility in information per se.

If there is an information argument in individuals' utility functions, it is easy to argue that it is likely to have greater weight in the context of screening than in, say, treatment programmes. However, while the weight attached to information may be less in treatment programmes, nonetheless it is likely to be present. In other words, and contrary to what is normally assumed in expected utility theory and in the QALY literature, information is likely to be present in the patient's utility function.

Autonomy and decision-making

Yet another argument in the patient's utility function relates to the issue of autonomy. Here, the word is used differently from the meaning implied in consumer sovereignty. With consumer sovereignty, economists tend to go beyond the basic idea that individuals are the best judges of their own welfare, and use consumer sovereignty to suggest that this applies to consumption choices. In other words, the fact of consumer sovereignty leads on to the idea that it is the individual's values that are to be used in consumption choices and that it is the consumer who is to make the consumption choices. Autonomy (which, interestingly, does not appear in my dictionary of economics) is defined as being a wider concept, which gives the individual not only the right to make the consumption choices but also the right not to make the consumption choices. This important distinction allows choice (and/or ability to pass choice to an agent) to enter as an argument in the consumer's utility function. Because of its reliance on consumer sovereignty, expected utility theory does not allow for choice as an argument in the utility function.

It is unfortunate that in the medical literature the word 'autonomy' has several meanings and that, in the wake of the move towards consumerism in health care, little thought seems to be given to whether the patient wants to exercise choice. In this context, there seems to be a strong argument for economists to analyse the medical literature on informed consent which, rather crudely, seems very often to be about doctor utility rather than patient utility. In other words, informed consent allows the doctor to shed some of the risk-bearing on to the patient with the result that the patient may suffer disutility not only from this increased risk-bearing but also from the receipt of the information per se. Here, ignorance on the part of the patient may be bliss and, under my proposed definition of autonomy, would be respected. Where autonomy moves in the direction of assuming that there must be utility in exercising informed choice, whatever the outcome and whatever the utility the patient derives from such choosing, then there is a departure from the way in which I am suggesting the concept of autonomy is used in the patient's utility function.

Process

Most of the economics literature on the topic of health care outputs is based on expected utility theory. Autonomy and decision-making are possible effects that may have an impact on individuals' utility but may be excluded under this theory. The theory is 'consequentialist' in the sense that it assumes that the only aspects of health care that have an impact on utility are outcomes and not processes – ends, in other words, and not means.

In practice, it can sometimes be quite difficult to sort out what is an outcome and what is a process. Here there is no need to debate whether it is necessary to create some new concept of process utility (although I would favour this). There is a need to widen research into health care outputs to include not just health and not just conventionally described outcomes. There are various processes that patients (and perhaps also citizens – see the discussion above on equity of access) undergo that may well be utility-bearing and that as such ought to be included in looking at the utility of health care services.

Deprivation

There is a literature in economics that considers various facets of utility beyond that of the conventional expected utility theory. It is suggested that there may well be legitimate reasons for doctors and others to want to reject QALYs when such QALYs are based solely on expected utility theory, as they tend to be in their current incarnation.

Let us look briefly at some of the arguments. First, QALYs normally assume that U(H1 − H2) = U(H1) − U(H2). In other words, QALYs, being expected utility theory based, assume that what is utility-bearing is states of the world and that the difference in utility in moving from state H1 to state H2 is the same as the numerical difference between the utility in state H1 and the utility in state H2. That seems questionable.

There is some evidence to support the view that the utility of a health state is not independent of the recent health state of the respondent, and it seems very likely that it would be a function of the current health state of the respondent. People appear to adjust to health states in the sense that the expected and realised utility may well vary as a result of some form of learning and/or coping process. Prospect theory can take this into account. There would seem to be much to be said for economists trying to work more with the sort of model that Kahneman and Tversky have developed under prospect theory.[9] (See Salkeld for one example.[10])

Here, regret theory is relevant.[11] Taking breast cancer screening as an example, when a breast screening opportunity arises, women who are deemed eligible can choose whether to be screened. Regret would arise if a woman chose not to be screened and then discovered subsequently that she had a breast cancer that could have been detected at an earlier stage if she had chosen to be screened. Here, one of the preconditions for the existence of regret is choice. The eligible woman made a personal choice not to be screened. She is worse off after choosing not to be screened than if the screening programme had not existed.

In the context of screening, six groups of women whose utility is potentially affected by access to a screening programme have been identified: the true and false positives and the true and false negatives (i.e. the women screened) and two other groups whose utility may be affected by the very existence of a screening programme.[12]

First, there are those women who, although eligible for screening, choose not to be screened and then suffer regret as a result of choosing not to take up the offer. Second are those women who are not eligible, and it is here that 'deprivation disutility' comes into play. It may be that such a screening programme is restricted to women over 50 and the under-50s feel deprived. Or, in the context of screening for Down's syndrome, a 34-year-old woman is not eligible because the cut-off point is 35 and only older women can be screened. Younger women, whatever the outcome of their pregnancy, may feel deprived and, even when their risk of giving birth to a Down's syndrome baby is unchanged, may suffer greater disutility than would be the case if the test for Down's syndrome did not exist at all. Of course, this assumes that the women know of the existence of the test and of their exclusion from it. It is important to note that, as compared with regret, deprivation does not involve choice on the part of the patient. Indeed, it is a precondition for the existence of deprivation disutility that the patient is deprived of choosing to have the service concerned.

This concept may be relevant in a number of areas of health care. Here, the decision context is something that economists appear not to take sufficient account of when discussing patients' utility functions and that the QALY literature ignores completely. For example, if a new technology is introduced, before it is disseminated widely it is likely that it will be restricted to a number of patients, perhaps in a particular geographical area. In this case, those who live elsewhere may suffer 'deprivation disutility' and be worse off than if the technology had never been introduced. (All of this assumes, of course, that these 'deprived' patients know of the existence of the technology.)

It follows that the existence of such disutility can be used as part of the reasoning for ensuring that access to this new technology is extended to all those potentially 'eligible', although this may not totally overcome the presence of deprivation disutility if the criterion for eligibility is based solely on some cost per QALY type of calculations. Again, much depends on the 'decision environment'.

Many hold the view that, if a particular form of treatment exists, then all who might benefit from it should have access to it. Birk, for example, found that of a sample of GP patients, over 90 per cent agreed or strongly agreed with the statement: 'If the public authorities sought to offer a test – for detecting cystic fibrosis – to anyone, then everyone in Denmark who wants it should have access to it.'[13] Clearly, such a view runs counter to the cost per QALY league table method of sorting out priorities. If applied, it would mean that, if societies had a particularly strong preference for such a criterion, then the question of which services to introduce, and when, would need to take more account of the eligibility criterion than is currently the case. It is, in a sense, a strong equity principle, yet it is not based on the same Margolis consideration for equity through participation discussed earlier in this chapter. Indeed, it is a much more selfishly based form of utility. It is the feeling on the part of an individual suffering from some problem that, since someone else is suffering from the same problem and is eligible for a particular form of treatment, then so should that individual. It is not that the first individual envies the second. It is perfectly possible that the concept of a 'caring externality', i.e. individuals care about others in some way or other, may operate here alongside that of deprivation disutility.

4.5 Conclusion

There are five conclusions that readers might draw from the series of thoughts and discussion in this chapter. First, health status measurement is difficult but possible and desirable. Second, there is no gold standard in how to do it. Third, economists need to do more work on attempting to find out rather than just assuming that we (along with doctors) already know what is in the patient's utility function. Fourth, there is a need to consider more carefully the decision environment in which any measures of output are to be used in economic evaluations. Both the arguments in the utility function and the weights attached to them may well be decision-specific. And fifth, the task is to measure what should be measured rather than measure and model something else because it is measured and modelled more readily. That is a fate that has befallen much of the work in equity. It seems important not to fall into the same trap when attempts are made to measure the outputs of the health care system.

Questions

1. How would you distinguish between ordinal and cardinal? Does the distinction matter in health status measurement?
2. How do ratio and interval scales differ?
3. Who is the father of QALYS?
4. What is the standard gamble?
5. What are the bare bones of the Margolis fair shares model?
6. Is information per se valuable?
7. What is autonomy? How does it differ from consumer sovereignty?
8. What is 'deprivation disutility'?

Notes

1. J. Dowie, 'Decision validity should determine whether a generic or condition specific HRQOL measure is used in health care decision making', *Health Economics*, 11 (2002), pp 1–8; 'Rejoinder', *Health Economics*, 11 (2002), pp 21–2.
2. G. Guyatt, 'Commentary on Jack Dowie', *Health Economics*, 11 (2002), pp 9–12.
3. D. Feeny, 'Commentary on Jack Dowie', *Health Economics*, 11 (2002), pp 13–16.
4. J. Brazier and R. Fitzpatrick, 'Measures of health related quality of life in an imperfect world', *Health Economics*, 11 (2000), pp 17–20.
5. G.W. Torrance, 'Social preferences for health states, and empirical evaluation of three measurement techniques', *Socio-Economic Planning Science*, 10 (1976), p 129.
6. A. Williams, 'Economics of coronary artery bypass grafting', *British Medical Journal*, 291, (1985), p 326.
7. H. Margolis, *Selfishness, Altruism and Rationality* (Cambridge University Press: Cambridge, 1982).
8. G. Mooney and M. Lange, 'Antenatal screening: what constitutes benefit?', *Social Science and Medicine*, 37 (1993), pp 873–878.
9. D. Kahnemann and A. Tversky, 'Prospect theory: an analysis of decision making under risk', *Econometrica*, 47 (1979), pp 263–291.

10. G. Salkeld, 'The nature of the maximand for preventive care', PhD Thesis (Department of Public Health, University of Sydney, 2001).
11. G. Loomes and R. Sugden, 'Regret theory: an alternative theory of rational choice under uncertainty', *Economic Journal*, 92 (1982), pp 805–824.
12. M. Lange, K. Gerard, D. Turnbull and G. Mooney, 'Economic evaluation of mammography screening: information, reassurance and anxiety', CHERE monograph (Department of Public Health, University of Sydney, 1994).
13. H. Birk, 'Udledning af byttefunktionen med hensyyn til sundhedsydleser, Stor opgave' [Development of a utility function for health services], Masters dissertation (Department of Economics, University of Copenhagen, 1995).

five

Values in health care

Somebody somewhere should explicitly decide who shall live and who shall die.

5.1 Whose values?

How do doctors decide? Indeed, what should doctors decide? There is room for improvement – and understanding – on how doctors make decisions. This point is not intended to be overly critical. It is to accept, however, that the extent to which individual doctors acting in the best interests of their patients – best as they see it – are or indeed should be involved in issues of efficiency and perhaps equity. What I want to concentrate on here is one aspect of this: the issue of valuation. First, we will consider the question of whose values; second, the question of how we elicit values from the relevant valuers; and lastly, the question of how we might 'best' proceed.

This is the area of health economics that is most disturbing for most health care professionals. To be trained in medicine, nursing or one of the other 'sharp-end' disciplines and then be faced with some hard-nosed, cold-blooded, pointy-headed economist placing money values on human life and suffering is anathema to many. Maybe it is no help to know that we have no choice as to whether we do this valuing; our only choice is whether to do it explicitly and thereby better or implicitly and almost certainly badly.

Let's get the issue of the inevitability of the process sorted out first. Returning to some of the basic principles of economics discussed in Chapter 2, if I decide to buy an avocado priced at £1, from this behaviour you can immediately tell that I value an avocado at at least £1, otherwise I wouldn't buy it. If, additionally, I refuse to buy an avocado when it is priced at £1.10, then you can judge that I value an avocado at between £1 and £1.10. Thus, faced with costs of consumption, our behaviour can tell observers quite a lot about the value we place on the benefits we get from our consumption. In other words, through these 'implied values' we reveal our preferences by our behaviour.

The same is true in principle in health care, even if it is not always the consumer who is doing the valuing. If a decision is made to spend £2 million on dialysis machines that have been estimated to result in an extra 100 years of life for patients treated but not to spend yet another £2 million, which would save another 50 years of life, then the implication is that the decision-maker is valuing a year of life on dialysis at at least £20,000 but not at £40,000. This is based on the simple premise that, if we say yes to a purchase, we can see what the implicit minimum value must be on the basis that benefits must be at least as great as the costs or we would not say yes. If we say no, that similarly places a maximum value on the purchase (or, strictly, the non-purchase).

Such decisions cannot be avoided; consequently, such valuing is inevitable. But even if it is inevitable, does that necessarily make it desirable that we attempt to make those values explicit? Death itself is inevitable – but, given the taboos that surround it, that does not mean that it is necessarily good for us to think about it explicitly, or at least not too often.

The example of the estimated values of life in different sectors of the economy is useful and is taken from Elvik,[1] who in turn based much of his analysis on Tengs et al.[2] Table 5.1 is reproduced from Elvik.

Table 5.1 Cost-effectiveness of 587 life-saving interventions

	Cost-effectiveness of life-saving interventions in 1993 (US dollars per life year gained)		
Sector of society	Median cost per life year gained	Minimum cost per life year gained	Maximum cost per life year gained
Medical ($n = 310$)	19,000	0	26,000,000
Residential ($n = 30$)	36,000	0	18,000,000
Transport ($n = 87$)	56,000	0	10,000,000
Occupational ($n = 36$)	350,000	0	99,000,000,000
Environmental ($n = 124$)	4,200,000	0	34,000,000,000
All sectors ($n = 587$)	42,000	0	99,000,000,000

Source: Elvik (2002); adapted from Tengs et al. (1995).

This is purely illustrative, but it gives an indication of how comparing the effectiveness of life-saving programmes in different sectors of the economy might allow judgements to be formed about the relative implied value of life in different sectors. Caution in interpreting these figures is immediately needed in that the mix of benefits (in terms of saved lives and at different ages, reduced morbidity, reduced injuries, etc.) might not be constant across the different sectors and the marginal cost per life saved might not follow the same pattern as the median values. Allowing for all of that, however, it is most likely that there is inefficiency in the allocation of scarce societal resources across the different sectors of the economy as revealed in Table 5.1.

What is being said here, in effect, is that making values explicit can by itself help to begin to get decision-makers to question whether they might be able to be more efficient or indeed be better at pursuing other objectives.

The issue in such examples is, given certain assumptions, spelled out as best one can, how does spending on life-saving in some area or another compare with the return on similar spending elsewhere? In other words, do we save more lives if we spend on environmental protection of the atmosphere or on road safety or health care?

The argument is that presenting such cost data and thereby implied values explicitly helps the decision-making process. It certainly does not make the decision. To do that requires consideration of the weight to be attached to economic efficiency (vis-à-vis, for example, equity), of the assumptions used and of whose values are to be deemed relevant in making the decisions.

The answer to the question of whose values to use in health care will depend on many factors. Prime among these are what type of health care system we are considering, what types of health care we are examining and why we are asking the question.

In 'normal' market economics, economists usually assume that the knowledgeable consumer is the one whose preferences are to count; that is, the concept of consumer sovereignty, as discussed in Chapter 2, applies. When we examine the markets for health care, as we discovered in Chapter 3, the situation in all countries, whatever the organising and financing of health care, looks rather different.

How relevant is consumer sovereignty in health care? Is conventional economic demand theory (as spelled out in Chapter 2) appropriate?

If consumer sovereignty is to apply, then three questions have to be answered in the affirmative:

1. Does the individual accept that they are the best person to judge their own welfare?
2. Is the individual able to judge their own welfare?
3. Does the individual want to make the appropriate judgement?

Let us look at these three questions in some detail. Question 1 essentially concerns whether the consumer believes in consumer sovereignty in principle in health care. This relates to the underlying ethics as seen by the consumer, an issue to be debated in Chapter 7. Or is the consumer more inclined to the view that their own preferences are so likely to be wrong that the principle of consumer sovereignty in the context of health care should be broken – indeed, that that is the very reason why we train a medical elite?

Going back to the discussion in Chapter 3 of the nature of health and health care and to our three questions on consumer sovereignty, it seems very likely that in health care the individual's manifest preferences and their true preferences will not be the same. It is thus the case that the separation of these two types of preference is very relevant in health care. I will discuss whether social welfare should be based on manifest preferences, under the question of whether the individual wants to make the appropriate judgements. Consequently, in answer to our first question I think we can safely say that the principle of autonomy should apply to the issue of whether the individual accepts consumer sovereignty for themselves or not. The answer to that question will very likely depend on the cultural and health care system setting in which it is posed.

Adopting this stance allows us to retain the economist's god of rationality. This notion simply involves adopting behaviour that allows us consistently to pursue our goals. Within this it is quite rational to argue as individuals that in principle the most rational stance for us to adopt on values in decision-making in health care is to accept that we are not well placed by ourselves to get our manifest preferences to coincide with our true preferences. We need help; we need an agent acting on our behalf.

But then, turning to our second question, is the individual able to judge their own welfare? Against the background of the discussion in Chapter 3, the answer here must surely be no in many situations.

Many individuals in many circumstances in health care have great difficulty in understanding what is wrong with their health. They are unlikely to know the effects of different forms of treatment, and even if they do they may not be able to evaluate the disutility of different health states. There may be some sort of continuum that stretches from conditions about which the relevant utility and disutility are very well known to the individual, to others about which they know little or nothing. This continuum may well be matched by one that reflects a complete ability to form the necessary judgements about the value of health care to complete lack of ability. This in turn will be reflected in a valuation system that stretches from the one pole of consumer sovereignty to the other of imposed 'merit goods'. (A 'merit good' embodies the notion that some elite is better placed than individuals to form judgements about what individuals' preferences ought to be.)

I think this provides a good idea of some of the problems in sticking too firmly to consumer sovereignty in health care. But it carries with it a problem in that it requires not only an ability to measure values under very different value bases but also an awareness of which and whose values apply to what policy questions and what level of mix is appropriate in differing circumstances.

There may be a similar but yet simpler answer to this issue. Given that society has invested substantial resources in educating doctors in such matters, the individual 'consumer' (i.e. patient) may simply opt out and leave most of this to the doctor. After all, is that not what the doctor is trained for? There has been a tendency in recent years to 'commodify' health care and to bring the language of the marketplace into this social service, including the use of expressions such as 'consumers' and 'customers', 'providers' and 'business plans'. It is just possible that many people who approach the health service when they are sick are happy to be 'patients'.

What about our third question, which we have already touched on in Chapter 3? It might seem that by answering the first we would have the answer to the third, but that does not necessarily follow. The process of choice may have a value in itself; the utility here can be a function of, for example, our belief in individual autonomy, our concern about getting decisions right (or failing to get them wrong) *additional* to the outcome of getting it right and our desire to blame others if the decision is wrong.

Freedom to choose does not necessarily have a positive utility attached to it. It may be negative. If I want to *not* make the decision ('Doctor, I can't decide. What do you think?'), to be forced to do so may diminish my utility, even if the outcome in terms of the impact on my health status remains the same. There is an important ethical issue here.

A related and potentially important issue is the question of what might be described as autonomous externalities. If I believe in freedom of choice for myself, this may influence my neighbour to believe similarly. Clearly, with many issues, my beliefs may influence my neighbour's and vice versa. But I would argue that, in the context of a principle such as this, it is often the case that as individuals we positively seek support for our principles in our neighbours, friends, colleagues, and so on.

But these autonomous externalities may take a less passive form. Crudely, this has been expressed in the political slogan 'people should stand on their own two feet'. The relevance to our discussion here is that this view is expressed about not just the speaker but about others, and indeed it is often directed specifically and explicitly at those who appear unwilling to accept this dictum. In other words, freedom of choice is deemed to be a good thing, regardless of whether individuals want to choose to have freedom of choice. (There are also equity considerations here, since one individual's ability to choose may well be different from another's – but that is another issue.)

Clearly, the value system on which any health care service is based is exceedingly complex and indeed constitutes potentially a series of systems that may vary across different services within health care and across different cultures and time periods. Thus, the basis on which we value health and health care is a cultural and changing phenomenon that cannot be – or at least ought not to be – seen in a vacuum, as it were, and separate from other concerns of governments and nations or indeed culture in its widest sense. For example, the issue of freedom of individual choice will be a more important driving force in some societies than in others, and in turn will be more important in some health care systems than in others.

In recent times, the move seems to have been to more and more consumer sovereignty in health care mixed with concern about promoting more and more efficiency. Unfortunately, these two are becoming confused and, indeed, in some people's minds, synonymous. This is unhelpful, particularly when the medical profession appears by and large to be part of the trend towards greater individual autonomy in health care. In fact, it may be leading it. Given that the profession is not neutral about the outcome of any great debate about health care and that it is a potent force within all health care systems, its attitudes, values and behaviour may be of paramount importance in determining the outcome. There can be little doubt, as three leading Canadian economists wrote a quarter of a century ago, but it remains as true today about values in health care: 'Providers hold the key to the dynamics of the health care market.'[3] It is at our peril – whether we are considering the supply side of the market or the demand side – that we ignore this fact.

5.2 Valuing outputs

To value outputs in health care is technically difficult; to defend doing so is morally easy. Most readers, in so far as they have thought about this issue at all, have perhaps had difficulty with the morality and glossed over the technical problems. As indicated, the explicit valuing of health outputs promotes economic efficiency, and economic efficiency promotes health. Morally, then, that position is defensible. (This should not be confused with the moral dilemma that it throws up: essentially, whether it is morally right that somebody, somewhere should *explicitly* decide who shall live and (the opportunity cost) who shall die. I am sympathetic to those health service decision-makers who worry about this issue. But the costs of avoiding it are too high. For those who do not like it, it may be that they need to be replaced by those more prepared to play the grizzly algebraic game of y chronic renal failure patients given x years' more life versus z cases of psoriasis treated successfully.)

It is not, however, central to this book that the reader has a detailed knowledge of how health outputs are valued. (For more information on this, see Donaldson[4] and Ryan and Farrar.[5]) Briefly, there are three methods commonly encountered. First, there is the implied-values approach already discussed. This has the merit of being based on the existing decision-making procedures and value structure of health care. Essentially, it teases out the values implied by past decisions. In so far as these emerge as being very different from one another, then for similar outputs at the margin of different programmes they can be used to examine whether some technical inefficiencies are present; that is, if the implied value of life in one program is £1 million and, for similar lives, in another it is £100,000, there is inefficiency present in that a shift of funds from the first programme to the second would result in an overall gain in lives saved. (Ideally, we want to move to the position where the marginal implied values of similar outputs are the same in all programmes.)

If the values that emerge for the same marginal output in different programmes are similar, then these may be used in evaluating new programmes that come up for examination. Unfortunately, little work has been done on this approach, but what has been done suggests that the implied values emerging, for values of life at least, vary markedly.

A second approach, and indeed that encountered most commonly, equates the value of life with the value of livelihood. This human capital approach suggests that people may be valued in terms of their productive output, the valuation of which is equated with their earnings (or, more accurately, the labour costs of employing them, which will usually be greater than earnings), discounted through time and adjusted to allow for expected participation in the labour force. In the context of health care, it may be argued that this at least provides 'floor' values since one objective of health care is to get people back to productive employment. In so far as there are other objectives, the value emerging has to be a minimum. Clearly, there are major problems with this omission of non-work values, particularly as it leaves the valuation of pensioners and many women at worst at zero and at best problematical. Perhaps its main virtues are its ease of applicability and the fact that it does allow relevant market outputs to be valued.

A third approach is that of consumer demand: essentially, attempting to determine how much individuals are prepared to pay to reduce their risk of death or morbidity from some existing low level to some still lower level. Thus individuals faced with a risk of death of, say, three in 1000 might be asked how much they would be prepared to pay to reduce this to two in 1000. If on average 1000 individuals said £200, then the 'value of life' would be £200,000 (i.e. £200 × 1000). This willingness to pay (WTP) approach is currently the one most fashionable among economists primarily because it satisfies their concern with consumer sovereignty. But then, given the discussion in Chapter 3 and earlier in this chapter, it is far from clear that consumer sovereignty based values – at least unadulterated ones – are appropriate in health care valuation.

What should we do in practice? Beyond attempting to improve the methodology of valuation, perhaps the most sensible approach at the present time is to adopt the implied-values method. It requires the least stretching of the health care decision-makers' imagination and credence, which, in the short run at least, is perhaps the best criterion to adopt. If economists wish to appear credible as analysts generally in health care, then in this particular arena a little cautious tiptoeing is justified.

What must be emphasised is that the issue cannot be avoided. That is the crucial message. It is a message that is explicitly spelled out in the implied-values approach. So, in the short run at least, perhaps we should leave it there, except to add that the emphasis placed on different value systems ought not to be treated as exogenous. *What* is to be valued – that is, what the objectives and outputs are – and *how* values are derived may be influenced by agents within health care. This broad issue is one we will return to in the last chapter of this book.

5.3 Que faire?

So what do we do about values, valuers and valuation in health care? The messages emerging from this chapter are simple. First, it is not for economists to determine what the bases of the value systems in health care should be or who the valuers should be, although we can point to the implications of different choices. Second, attempting to determine what these bases are is important, and economics can help with that. Third, whatever the bases, making the values in decision-making explicit can only be good for any health service – good in the sense of leading to increased efficiency and other objectives. Again, economics can clearly assist with this.

Too often it seems that health service decision-makers are not aware of the extent to which value judgements enter into their decision-making. Additionally, it would seem important to provoke a debate about the appropriateness of different actors' value judgements at different levels of decision-making. Perhaps this chapter has helped to highlight some of the issues here. The next chapter takes the process further and suggests how some of the different values can be partially reconciled.

This issue is returned to in the final chapter, but there I come off the fence and argue for community values in at least setting the principles on which health care systems should be based.

Questions

1. Whose values in health care?
2. Whose values in 'normal' markets?
3. What is consumer sovereignty?
4. What is a 'merit good'? Give examples.
5. Is freedom to choose always a good thing?
6. What is the 'human capital' value of life?

Notes

1. R. Elvik, 'Cost–benefit analysis of ambulance and rescue helicopters in Norway', *Applied Health Economics and Health Policy*, 1 (2002), pp 5–13.
2. T.O. Tengs, M.E. Adams, J.E. Pliskin, et al., 'Five hundred life saving interventions and their cost-effectiveness', *Risk Analysis*, 15 (1995), pp 369–390.
3. M.L. Barer, R.G. Evans and G.L. Stoddart, *Controlling for Health Care Costs by Direct Charges to Patients: Snare or Delusion?* (Ontario Economic Council: Toronto, 1979).
4. C. Donaldson, 'Eliciting patients' values by use of willingness to pay', *Health Expectations*, 4 (2001), pp 180–188.
5. M. Ryan and S. Farrar, 'Using conjoint analysis to elicit preferences for health care', *British Medical Journal*, 320 (2000), pp 1530.

six

Need, demand and the agency relationship

Maybe we don't need demand but should we demand need?

6.1 Introduction

The concept of demand was discussed in Chapter 2 and that of need was mentioned in Chapter 3. In this chapter, some of the key elements of demand and need and the relationship (where it exists) between them are highlighted. There is a now vast and still expanding literature on this broad area, and it is not intended for any sort of comprehensive survey of existing research to be presented. Rather, some aspects that were raised earlier are now brought together.

Economists, as the reader will now be aware, are wont to argue that the issue of values in health care is of major importance. Further, they suggest that the criteria for choosing which 'actors' perform which 'roles' in the valuation process ought to be made much more explicit than is often the case in current health service decision-making. Indeed, it is possible in this book to introduce the reader to only a little of the material written about the nature of the commodities health and health care, about the problems of market failure, about the extent to which any conventional economic theory of demand is relevant to health care, about the nature and relevance of the concept of need, and the role, in theory at least, of the agency relationship in health care supply and demand. For those who wish to pursue this particular topic in more detail, Arrow,[1] McGuire et al.[2] and Rice[3] are especially recommended.

6.2 Demand and the need for health care

As was discussed in Chapter 2, economists tend to assume in the context of conventional demand theory that consumers are well informed and able and willing to make their own decisions regarding their consumption behaviour. In other words, the sovereign consumer chooses to exercise their sovereignty by making explicit, rational choices between different goods and services in order to maximise their utility. Given the nature of health care (as outlined in Chapter 3) and the question mark raised about the role of consumers' preferences in Chapter 5, there have to be some doubts about the relevance of conventional demand theory in health care. In particular, uncertainty and lack of information are likely to create difficulties in applying demand theory in an unadulterated form to the commodity of health care. But this does not mean that demand is of no assistance in analysing health care. What needs to be resolved is the debate in Chapter 5. In other words, what is the extent and nature of the departure needed from conventional demand theory in the health care sector?

Grossman, whose ideas were aired in Chapter 3 and have influenced much of the thinking of health economists in the last 30 years (although perhaps not so much of late), argues that consumers do have enough information to be able to make rational choices about their health both currently and in the future.[4] Grossman suggests that the individual's demand for health care is derived from their perception of their optimal level of health. The demand for health care consequently arises because the individual wants to bridge the gap between their perceived current health state and some higher health state that they desire. As a result of this desire, one course of action – others are clearly possible – is for the individual to decide to seek health care.

At the other end of the spectrum, it is possible to view the consumer as being much less knowledgeable than Grossman assumes. The consumer may be ignorant about both current and future health states, the range and effectiveness of treatments available, and so on. In such a view of the patient's position, it is the doctor who both supplies the information necessary to make rational choices and makes the decision about which treatment and to what extent is required for the particular health state of the patient, as diagnosed by the doctor.

This 'needs' approach is based on the notion of 'merit goods', introduced in Chapter 5, and reflects the judgements of some elite – in this case, medical doctors who either impose their judgements on the patients or have their decisions accepted by the patients. (The jargon of 'merit goods' has come in for some justified cynicism from one economist, Margolis, who suggests that a merit good is 'any item of public expenditure that seems socially reasonable but cannot be accounted for within the ordinary economic theory of demand. It is a kind of formalised escape clause'.[5])

Clearly, the concept of need conflicts with that of consumer sovereignty. Yet it would be wrong to place consumer sovereignty on a pedestal. There will be occasions when some correction or even replacement of ignorant consumers' preferences will be justified. Certainly, as Chapter 5 indicated, there has to be some debate about who should formulate the relevant valuations. In practice in health care, need does creep in but seldom to the complete exclusion of demand.

It can also be argued that the need for health services is a function of the need for health per se. In a sense, this is self-evident. Yet in much of the debate about 'need', this simple notion of the need for health care being a 'derived' need – that is, derived from the need for health – tends to be lost sight of.

One thing that clearly emerges from the different views of 'need' is that, in using the word, we must be very careful to convey precisely what it is that we mean. Indeed, in some debates about health care policy, one is occasionally left with the feeling that use of the word 'need' is designed deliberately to confuse the listener and to stifle rational thought and debate. ('We *need* a new hospital': end of story.) For economists, need is an evaluative, normative notion that has some kind of objective lying behind it.

It is all too easy in considering need to assume that, if a treatable condition exists, (1) it should be treated and (2) it should be treated in the best way possible, 'best' here being defined as 'medically most effective'. If this were accepted, this would mean that all need should be treated and only the most effective treatments should be used. Both of these ignore the facts that resources are scarce and an overall better use of resources may be obtained from employing less effective but cheaper policies.

Doubts about the relevance of demand lead to the view that ideas of value (and hence of need) may be more suitably elicited from people other than the consumers themselves. This is part of the reason why, in health economics, we might prefer to talk about a 'marginal value curve' rather than a demand curve. Indeed at one International Health Economics Association (the 'world body of health economics') conference there was a debate about whether the demand curve exists at all in health care. With a demand curve, it is assumed that the consumers are doing the valuation (i.e. consumer sovereignty is operating). In the case of a marginal value curve, the question of who is doing the valuing is left open. If it is the consumers, then the demand curve and the marginal value curve are synonymous. In practice, since the commodity of health care is not homogeneous – a consultation with a general practitioner is very different from treatment in intensive care – the degree to which need or demand is appropriate will tend to vary with the service being discussed.

In any debate about total need, what has to be emphasised is that not all need can be met and that there will be a ranking of needs in the sense that, *ceteris paribus*, we would prefer one need to be met rather than another (e.g. if the former yielded a higher benefit than the latter). But the *ceteris paribus* assumption may not hold. In particular, it may not hold with regard to cost. Given the concept of opportunity cost, clearly it is the case that the choice of what needs to meet should be in part a function of the costs involved – and that, in meeting need, it is not necessarily the most effective mechanism that should be adopted. Further, the extent to which particular needs are to be met will again be a function of both benefits and costs of doing so, strictly marginal costs and marginal benefits. Need is not absolute and finite. It is dynamic and tends to grow through time – and of particular interest, its growth is at least in part a function of the growth in supply of health care facilities.

Maybe the sentiments expressed in the last paragraph are the most important in the book. Certainly I believe they are true. More importantly, so many decision-makers in health care seem not to believe that they are true or at least act as if they are not true. Need is so often driven by epidemiologists, yet as one eminent epidemiologist, Kawachi, has written, 'Epidemiology is the science of counting.'[6] If any concept in health care planning and policy-making needs more thought, it is need. Yes, quantification and measurement matter, but first let's think through what we want to measure and in particular sort out the value base of need.

It is important, in the context of values, that the morality of recognising that need is not absolute and cannot be met in full is accepted.

This form of need is in terms of 'capacity to benefit'. This idea from Culyer[7] has not taken off in health policy to the extent that it might have. (It is discussed in more detail in Chapter 8.) Some health problems are more amenable to health care interventions than others. Some problems, in other words, have a greater capacity to benefit from health care interventions than others.

In so far as health care policy-makers seem at times somewhat obsessed with the size of the problems (e.g. see Murray et al.[8] and for a response see Wiseman and Mooney[9]), the emphasis in this form of need is more on the size of the solution. 'What good can be done?' seems like a legitimate question to pose when allocating scarce health care resources. 'What good can be done by spending here rather than there?' seems an even more relevant question. Too often, it seems, big problems rather than best buys dominate. Faced with a limited health care budget, best buys should win all the time.

This of course raises the questions 'What is best?' and 'Who decides what is best?' What is most important is that these questions get asked. The 'big problems' answer is the unthinking answer to a question that does not get asked but is assumed. 'Big problems' is, in economic terms, also the wrong answer. It is most unlikely to promote efficiency and, with respect to equity, as will be demonstrated in Chapter 9, it is unlikely to deliver that either (although it may have more of a role here).

The central implication of all this is that the cost–benefit approach, which is essentially the weighing-up of costs – opportunity costs – and benefits, offers the most comprehensive method of coping with the problems raised in devising and using social indicators and measuring and using the concept of need. It is important to try to pick up the general principles involved:

- There is an opportunity cost of producing more health, for example in education benefits foregone.
- Some possible combinations of health and education will be preferred to others.
- What is sought is to obtain the most preferred combination from the resources available.
- Improved technology/increased productivity in the health care sector will not necessarily lead to any freed resources all being spent on health.
- Generally, the concept of need is useful if it is couched in cost–benefit terms, where trade-offs are made explicit.
- Generally, the concept of need set in terms of big problems is unhelpful to resource allocation for efficiency and only sometimes for equity.

If the reader can see their way to grasping these points, then that is sufficient for the purposes of this book. Certainly, the concept of need is difficult. Consequently, it may be helpful to summarise some key ideas about it:

- There is a lot of confusion and illogical thinking about and surrounding the concept of need, sometimes perhaps deliberate in an attempt to stifle debate.
- Need ought not to be determined without considering what the end is that is being sought and to which the services in question are instrumental means.
- Ignoring the possibilities for substitutability in meeting needs is likely to lead to problems and breed inefficiency.
- Almost always, no matter how need is defined, it embraces the idea of some third party being involved in the valuing process – unlike demand, where it is the consumer who is sovereign.
- *Which* third party is relevant, and *which* decisions are the key questions in the need/demand debate.
- Need is not absolute.
- Needs have to be ranked and should be costed.
- The particular contribution of economics to 'needology' derives from the proposition that the degree to which any given need will be met will depend upon the costs and benefits of meeting it.

The concepts of both demand and need are potentially of assistance in analysing and evaluating health care policy and, more importantly, the implications of different patterns of health care. The concept of demand retains the basic feature of the individual's own assessment of benefits. On the other hand, the concept of need, provided it encompasses some assessment of effectiveness, the potential for considering alternative ways of meeting need and to differing extents, and acceptance of resource constraints, can also form the basis for resource allocation. It will normally be best for both need and demand to be taken into account when a particular operation of a health service is being examined; neither demand nor need by itself is likely to provide a sufficient basis for decision-making. Unless an effort is made, first to resolve the issue of the sometimes conflicting values on the benefit side and then to incorporate relevant information on costs, resource allocation in health care is likely to remain less efficient than it otherwise might be.

6.3 Describing the agency relationship

The relationship between demand and need is clearly a complicated one. It can be argued that:

- As individuals, we all frequently have wants for better health.
- Some of these wants we do nothing about; for others, we actively seek health care (e.g. we attend a GP's surgery).
- The medical practitioner may not agree with us in our assessment of either wants or demands; some of our wants or demands, they may argue, do not need treatment, or there may be certain aspects of better health that we have not included in our wants or demands that the medical practitioner believes should be treated.

Need may be:

- demanded and wanted
- undemanded and wanted
- undemanded and unwanted.

Demanded and wanted needs are likely to have a higher value in the minds of patients than undemanded and wanted needs (presuming that it is the higher-priority wants that are more likely to be expressed as demand). They may not be perceived as being of higher value by the medical practitioner. Undemanded and unwanted needs are likely to have a lower value (indeed, they are of zero value in their current state of knowledge) in the minds of patients than either demanded, wanted needs or undemanded, wanted needs, but again this will not necessarily be the case for the medical practitioner. Indeed, without empirical data we have no way of ranking the priority that the medical practitioner will attach to the three types of need. The same case from a medical viewpoint could fall into each of the three types. For example, a woman with a malignant neoplasm of the breast might be any of the following:

- She may want treatment but, not realising how important it is to be treated, not bother to go to her GP (wanted, undemanded need).

- She may want treatment, demand it, and get it because the GP agrees that treatment is needed (wanted, demanded need).
- She may not want or demand treatment because she does not realise anything is wrong (unwanted, undemanded need).

Can need and demand be reconciled? One way of doing so is through the agency relationship, in which the better-informed doctor acts as the agent of the ill-informed patient. Such a relationship exists largely because of the information problems identified in Chapter 3, leading to the view that it is the doctor rather than the patient who frequently does the demanding.

For the relationship to operate efficiently, various information is required: (1) basic medical information, which usually is the sole province of the medical doctor; (2) background non-medical information (such as the patient's family circumstances, financial circumstances, etc.), which is more the province of the patient; and (3) the patient's preferences for both medical and non-medical issues (pain and discomfort, having to wait, etc.), which again tend to be more in the patient's domain.

It thus becomes clear that, while the agency relationship is important, it will work well only if the doctor is prepared to spend time and effort getting information about points (2) and (3) out of the patient and the patient is prepared to give the doctor information about points (2) and (3). If it is the patient who is to make the decision, it is also necessary for the doctor to give the patient the information in point (1) and for the patient to understand it enough to be able to turn it into knowledge.

In essence, what we have here is an attempt through the agency relationship to improve on the cost–benefit calculus that the patient would otherwise have to make. Consumption choices normally involve the consumer in weighing up the costs and benefits involved and then making a decision. Problems arise in health care because the consumer will normally not bear all the costs (because of third-party financing). The consumer may also have poor perception of those costs that he or she will have to bear, will have little information about the benefits he or she is likely to receive from different courses of action, and in such circumstances may be loathe to take on the responsibility of decision-making. The agency relationship then acts as a process to bring together the cost-bearing, benefit-receiving and decision-making aspects of the cost–benefit calculus.

It is easy to recognise that to have a perfect agency relationship is far from straightforward. The doctor will be well placed to judge the effectiveness of different forms of care, but may find it more difficult to judge the relative benefit to the patient of such effectiveness. More problematic still will be the estimation of costs by the doctor, not only of those falling on the patient but more generally. Add in a fee-per-item of service system of remuneration for doctors and the difficulties are compounded since the doctor's financial interests are then embodied directly in the decision-making process.

Beyond this individual patient–doctor agency relationship, there is the wider (and not wholly separate) agency relationship that the doctor (or perhaps clinical team) operates on behalf of the group of patients for which the doctor or the clinical team is responsible. Here, the doctor has to weigh up the benefits to the various patients involved or potentially involved when he or she cannot treat all (or at least not all) as well as he or she ideally might. One patient's benefits is another patient's benefits foregone. Here, the agency relationship has become concerned with priorities within the group. This raises important issues about whose values should count, who decides what is benefit, who decides what is best. The ground moves from patient care to social issues and, indeed, social priorities. In turn, that raises the question yet again of whose values are relevant to which situations (more about this in Chapter 7).

6.4 Analysing the agency relationship

With respect to financing in health care, under any health care system two of the most important considerations that arise in the context of agency are patient payment (how and how much the patient pays) and doctor payment (how and how much the doctor gets paid). Recognising these issues but not actually dealing with them in this section, I want to look more analytically at the agency relationship. This means that we need to look very closely at the factors that influence the behaviour of the actors (primarily the medical doctors and the patients) in this agency relationship.

There is, to my way of thinking, something of a paradox here. The agency relationship exists because of the presence of asymmetry of information in the health care market. The perfect agency relationship assumes that at no cost (at least to the patient) perfect information or at least as good information as the doctor has can be made available to the patient – and the patient then exercises consumer sovereignty. Yet it may be better to consider the agency relationship in terms not of perfection (of either it itself or information) but rather 'completeness' (where information is optimal in terms of its costs and benefits). That, of course, raises questions of costs to whom and benefits to whom.

Let us consider the agency relationship in another way, starting not from attempts to overcome the problems of asymmetry of information but rather from the standpoint of the individual patient attempting to maximise their utility.

Seen from this perspective, the role of the perfect agency may be viewed as assisting the patient to make the optimal consumption decisions, which presumably can be interpreted as assisting the patient to maximise utility. This will include (presumably) anything that the consumer wants as an argument in that utility function and may include not only improved health status but also the utility of reduced uncertainty, of avoiding difficult decisions or of retaining one's autonomy and perhaps of information (or ignorance) itself. It will also include the disutility of health care consumption not only in terms of patient time but also the anxiety, discomfort and inconvenience associated with being a patient.

It is difficult to specify all the potential arguments in the patient's utility function but that is not necessary when viewing the agency relationship from this perspective. The point in principle is that it is whatever is in that utility function when the patient 'demands' health care that is relevant.

Let us take the specific example of a DNA probe to indicate to women at risk whether their fetus is carrying a diseased gene that will lead to autosomal dominant polycystic kidney disease creating problems in adulthood. Adults, both men and women, who are themselves carriers, have a 50% chance of passing the disease on to a fetus. In most countries, women can choose to terminate the pregnancy if the fetus is affected. The test is not 100% accurate (but it is close to it).

Now, if such screening could be conducted without the woman knowing, then with respect to polycystic kidney disease the woman's agent could then present the woman with the information. The woman could then make an informed decision. But there are costs involved in the process of screening, and these should be considered in deciding on the optimal screening policy and weighed against their benefits in making a decision.

Let us assume that no woman chooses to abort as a result of having received the information. Health (neither of the woman nor of the fetus) is not affected so there is no health gain. Where anything the patient wants is considered as an argument in the patient's utility function, then that is the utility function to be used.

Before doing so, however, it is perhaps important to indicate that I have reservations about the value of considering a 'perfect' agency relationship. That might involve a desire to get back to (or advance to?) a neoclassical world of perfect information. More tenable, I believe, is an analysis of the agency relationship that never considers perfection but rather proposes two things: (1) that the patient's utility function as perceived by both the patient and the doctor/agent contains arguments related to the presence of the agent in the market, e.g. information and decision-making; and (2) that arguments in the patient's utility function also enter the doctor/agent's utility function.

Maybe all this goes to show is that we are dealing here with a complex phenomenon. Briefly, a Finnish study is relevant here. Holli and Hakama report that, for their study in Tampere of breast cancer patients close to death, there was a tendency to treat and investigate more intensively than might have been expected at that terminal stage: 'more attention was being paid to the cancer than to the patient'.[10]

What is interesting, thereafter, was that, after the publication of the first study showing the results to support these conclusions, the clinicians involved changed their behaviour.[11] They treated and diagnosed less in a subsequent but comparable cohort and were more involved in palliative care.

This is, I believe, a highly relevant story for health economics. It raises various questions. Did the patients' utility functions change between the two studies? Or was it solely the doctor's/agent's perceptions of them that changed? What are clinical doctors' objectives vis-à-vis their patients and to what extent are doctors trying to act as agents for their patients – in any of the senses raised above?

All the discussion to date has considered the agency relationship as it relates to the doctor/patient position. But it can also be argued that the doctor has a role as society's agent. Here we could debate at length the 'has' and 'ought to have' question. What seems particularly relevant is that there have to be difficulties for the medical doctor in maximising patient anything (health, utility or whatever) and maximising social welfare (however this is defined). It may be that some of these difficulties at least can be overcome by providing the right organisational and ethical environment where, with appropriate incentives, some appropriate mix of these agency roles can be attained.

Regardless of whether they succeed, the idea of the individual doctor/individual patient agency relationship seems sound as a basis for describing how most clinical doctors see their role. It is the basis of much in medical ethics today. The individual consumer of health care is badly placed to perform their own cost–benefit calculus and looks to the doctor for help. While one can argue that most doctors are not trained adequately to assess such benefits and costs (especially the latter), in my experience many clinicians will tend to agree that what they are trying to do is to perform this role.

What seems today to be the pertinent question is the extent to which this role can be combined with the role of agent for society and who should perform this latter role. I have very great doubts about the nature of the distribution of property rights in health care that would be required for the clinician to be given the task of combining these two often conflicting and incompatible roles.

That is not to say that policy should concentrate on ensuring that doctors perform their agency role well on behalf of their individual patients. Nor would I advocate ignoring the doctor's potential role in the pursuit of social efficiency. The goal here is to maintain the optimal agency relationship (between doctor and patient) that is conducive with maximising social welfare. That is probably the central task of health economics.

Without the 'conducive with maximising social welfare' qualification, the pursuit of efficiency becomes impossible since individual doctors pursuing the maximisation of their patients' utilities will not lead to the maximisation of social welfare. Additionally, of course, there is the risk that, if policy is not aimed at ensuring that the doctor/agent perceives the patient's maximand in terms of utility (as defined by the patient), then even the agency relationship at the individual patient level will not be optimal.

There is something about this agency relationship that really makes it so important in health economics. But since it is in many ways a partial replacement or surrogate for prices in a normal market, it is hardly surprising that it is important.

Questions

1. How do demand and need differ? Which is better?
2. Why is there an agency relationship in health care?
3. Is Grossman's theory sensible?
4. How should we decide which needs to meet?
5. Which is 'the science of counting'?
6. Who decides what is best?
7. Is need absolute?
8. What's the moral of the Tampere tale?

Notes

1. K.J. Arrow, 'Uncertainty and the welfare economies of medical care', *American Economic Review*, 53 (1963) pp 941–973.
2. A. McGuire, J. Henderson and G. Mooney *The Economics of Health Care* (Routledge and Kegan Paul: London, 1988).
3. T. Rice, *The Economics of Health Care Reconsidered*, second edition (Health Administration Press: Chicago, Illinois, 2002).
4. M. Grossman, 'On the concept of health capital and the demand for health', *Journal of Political Economy*, 80 (1972), pp 223–225.
5. H. Margolis, *Selfishness, Altruism and Rationality* (Cambridge University Press: Cambridge, 1982).
6. I. Kawachi, 'Social epidemiology', *Social Science and Medicine*, 54 (2002), pp 1739–1742.
7. A.J. Culyer, 'Health, health expenditures and equity', discussion paper 83 (Centre for Health Economics, University of York, York, 1991).
8. C. Murray, A. Lopez and D. Jamison, 'The global burden of disease', *Bulletin of the World Health Organization*, 72 (1994), pp 495–509.
9. V. Wiseman and G. Mooney, 'Burden of disease and priority setting', *Health Economics*, 9 (2000), pp 369–372.
10. K. Holli and M. Hakama, 'Treatment of the terminal stages of breast cancer', *British Medical Journal*, 31 (1989), pp 13–14.
11. K. Holli, M. Hakama and G. Mooney, 'Changing clinical practice, a case study in breast cancer'. In *Changing Values in Medical and Health Care Decision Making*, eds U.J. Jensen and G. Mooney (Wiley: London, 1990).

seven

The inefficiency of medical ethics

A doctor's got to do, what a doctor's got to do.
(with apologies to the late – and great – John Wayne)

7.1 Introduction

I have been intrigued for some years by the apparent concern about economics exhibited by many members of the medical profession. There is something about the two disciplines that makes economics and medicine difficult bedfellows. It cannot be that they share a lot of common ground, which is perhaps the rather crude explanation as to why there tend to be tensions between economists and accountants. Nor is it that economists and medical doctors are in some kind of power struggle, as seems so often the case with doctors and nurses. So why?

I think the answer may lie in the different ethical bases on which the two disciplines are founded. Certainly, medical ethics is important to the medical profession and to health care. Any threat to medical ethics seems capable of being interpreted as a threat to the professional status of doctors and perhaps even to their professional integrity. It is these and related issues that I want to discuss in this chapter.

In the wider context of the overall objectives of this book, I want to make a few observations from an economist's standpoint on the subject and practice of medical ethics. In particular, I want to highlight the uncomfortable fact that, as practised, medical ethics, particularly in the form of clinical freedom, tends to breed inefficiency. Indeed, it seems that it sometimes provides a convenient escape mechanism for the members of the medical profession neither to pursue efficiency nor to attempt any rationalisation at all of the potential for pursuing efficiency in health care.

Certainly, there are problems in applying economic analysis in health care, particularly in placing money values on the outputs (as we have seen already from Chapter 5). Given scarcity, however, we cannot avoid valuing human life.

The nub of the issue as I see it is this: It is not a question of ethics *or* economics. Ethics is about choice; but then so is economics. Without a wider use of economics in health care, inefficiencies will abound and decisions will be made less explicitly and hence less rationally than is desirable: we will go on spending large sums to save life in one way when similar lives in greater numbers could be saved in another way. The price of inefficiency, inexplicitness and irrationality in health care is paid in death and sickness.

Are things getting better? Recently, there has been much more discussion of economic issues in health care. Many medical doctors are today ready to accept the need for resource constraints. Yet the emphasis in medicine remains on the individual patient or at best on the group of patients for whom an individual doctor is responsible. The emphasis also remains on what doctors think health is and what they think patients want from their doctor. The extent to which there has been a shift in the values underpinning health care is, I believe, minimal. This is clearly an ethical issue even if the ethical focus has perhaps moved somewhat in the past 20 years. The issue of *whose* values has always been a major issue in health care policy-making. It remains a key issue today. In health economics, it is also the case that there is growing recognition that it is a key issue and indeed that economists may have some responsibility to address it. That is new.

7.2 Ethics and medical ethics

There are three principal theories of ethics: the ethics of virtue, of duty and of the common good. The first two are essentially individualistic ethics and the last social ethics. The ethical goal of economics is efficiency, which is a social goal – essentially, maximising the benefit (however defined) to society at large from the resources available (however constrained).

Clearly, in medicine there are problems: first, in determining what is the common good and, second, in devising appropriate institutional arrangements to allow it to prosper alongside the individual ethics of virtue and duty. There is what amounts to a serious lacuna in medical ethics. The health care industry is, in all developed countries, a major social service, with important (and varying) institutional arrangements where the quality and appropriateness of both health care and the institution are subject to political and public debate. Yet the medical profession holds to codes of ethics that do not take this into account adequately. Instead of recognising the hole, it would seem to want to paper it over with the other two doctrines of ethics: virtue and duty. Thus, clinical freedom – part of an *individual* ethic – is sometimes used to try to defend what could only be truly defensible on the basis of some ethic of the common good.

The main reason for the existence of medical ethics lies in the nature of health care, as discussed in Chapter 3. In particular, the asymmetry of information and the knowledge of the asymmetry of information between doctor and patient are critical. For 'normal' goods and services – books, concerts, lawnmowers – the individual is faced with a range of products about which they have various pieces of information concerning the utility they are likely to derive from them. Of course, it is not always the case that the expected utility/satisfaction (the basis of all consumer decisions) will equate with realised utility/satisfaction. (My avocado may turn out to be hard or rotten. But at least I will *know* when this occurs, and it may influence my future consumption pattern.)

Let us switch for a moment, however, to even wider considerations. It can be argued that the philosophy of utilitarianism is the political basis of most Western democracies. One of the apparent difficulties of utilitarianism is that it can be interpreted as being so much based on an individual ethic as to allow individuals (1) to do themselves harm and (2) to do so because of lack of appropriate information. The idea of maximising utility, the aim of utilitarianism and so dear to the hearts of many economists, has a very attractive ring to it – particularly when it is based on the idea of consumer sovereignty. Thus, the values underlying utilitarianism are usually seen as those of individuals.

As normally conceived, there are two aspects to utilitarianism: (1) individual, consumer sovereignty and (2) emphasis on utility being derived from what the individual receives. Given the nature of health care and what has been said about asymmetry of information, it would appear that we have a problem, should we wish to defend utilitarianism in medicine.

Harsanyi indicates that it is necessary 'to distinguish between a person's manifest preferences and his true preferences ... the latter being those ... he would have if he had all the relevant factual information, always reasoned with the greatest possible care and were in a state of mind most conducive to rational choice'.[1] The dangers of not adopting this stance are all too apparent; as Sen and Williams say, 'If people do not, in fact, get round to actually wanting what ... it would be rational for them to want, people may always be actually unsatisfied by the results of the correct policy.'[2]

Much but not all of this is summed up by Amartya Sen, who writes that not everyone has an adequate capacity to manage to desire.[3] While this is less likely to be the case with avocados than with health care, and indeed would seem to matter less with such objects of consumption, in health care this notion of a patient's inability to manage to desire adequately seems rather important.

Clearly, in health care there are very real problems for individuals in assessing their true preferences. It is this issue that is crucial to valuation in health care and, consequently, to the potential usefulness of utilitarianism in health care decision-making.

For the doctor to act to bridge the gap between the patient's manifest and true preferences (as disclosed in Chapter 6), it is not enough for the doctor to consider what is prudent in *health* terms for their patient, were that patient as informed as the doctor. In pursuing what the doctor considers prudent, there will be some costs that will fall on the patient and that need to be assessed from the patient's point of view as if the patient were prudent. What is the cost *to the patient* of their time off work or their loss of time spent jogging – as judged by the doctor – assuming the patient were to act in a reasonably informed way? There will clearly also be costs to the doctor, which will mean that this agency relationship will be, at best, incomplete. Additionally, there is plenty of evidence to indicate that doctors do not know best when assessing a patient's quality of life.

There is a problem here that is important for medical ethics. While we (as patients and potential patients) may be prepared to accept that the doctor knows best when assessing health benefits, when it comes to weighing them against costs (of time, inconvenience, etc.) in the cost–benefit calculus, can we be as certain that the doctor can estimate accurately such costs from the perspective of the prudent patient?

There is, however, a second difficulty here (raised initially in Chapter 5), and that is that utilitarianism is often based on the idea of utility being derived *solely* from what is obtained (i.e. 'outcome' utility). This is disputed by some utilitarians, particularly on the issue of the utility derived from freedom of choice. It can readily be argued that utility may depend not only on what one gets but also on how one gets it.

There is the issue here of the utility of freedom of choice. Indeed, it is possible to take the view that, even if an individual were to do themselves harm and, after the event, know that they had done so because they had acted on the basis of poor information, nonetheless the individual would have been resentful (suffered disutility?) if someone had interfered with their freedom of choice.

Fortunately, and sensibly, there is a middle ground – not born of the desire for compromise per se but rather perfectly rational – within the utilitarian goal of maximising utility. It can be argued that, if people derive utility (positive or negative) from the process through which they receive a particular outcome, then that 'process' utility is relevant in deciding on how that person's overall utility is maximised. If this is the case (and it seems intuitively likely), then it is clearly not enough to consider *outcome* utility alone.

Many have defended the concept of greater freedom of choice for consumers in health care. Indeed, all private health care might be argued to be based on this idea of freedom. But the decision on whether to opt for greater freedom of choice hinges not solely on the utility associated with that freedom (assuming it is positive) but also on the overall utility, including outcome utility, in the two situations of less (public) or more (private) freedom of choice. Given the very real problems (particularly of ignorance) for individuals in exercising choice in health care, freedom of choice may have a negative utility. Thus, process utility in a public health care system may be positive, and individual freedom of choice may have an overall negative process utility.

For the present, I want to suggest that medical ethics has a potential impact on utility in the context not only of outcome utility (i.e. that through the existence of an ethical code the consumer can be reassured that the doctor's recommendations for action can be equated with the way in which the patient would act were they perfectly prudent) but also of process utility (i.e. the nature of the delivery and organisation of health care). Thus, individual ethics (virtue and duty) and collective ethics (the common good) can influence *how* the patient receives treatment. Indeed, the nature of the patient's demand for health care may well be, in part, a function of the nature and role of medical ethics in the health care system.

This comment on demand leads on to consideration of why doctors seek a medical ethic within which to operate. It can breed self-regulation when outside or external regulation might be either difficult or costly. Doctors can be reassured that they are working within reasonable guidelines if they stick to the ethical code, particularly given the nature and extent of medical practice variations. Doctors do make mistakes sometimes. If, however, they have followed medical ethical codes, then there is likely to be less moral comeback.

Thirdly, the introduction of ethics will shift the demand curve for medical care outwards (the quantity demanded of ethical care will be greater than that of 'unethical' care, all other things being equal). Thus, there may be pecuniary reasons for ethics where quantity demanded affects doctor remuneration. Essentially, therefore, there are both supply-side and demand-side arguments for medical ethics. To couch the issue in these 'market'-oriented terms may also be very appropriate since medical ethics, as distinct from health care ethics, is restricted largely to the individual ethics of virtue and duty.

The problem for the medical profession, and indeed all of us, is that much of medical ethics is the product of another time when medicine and the market had a much closer affinity. With the complexity of modern health care systems and the increased concern and involvement of governments in health services, the individualistic ethics of the medical profession need to be harnessed to (but not replaced by) an ethic of the common good. The 'invisible hand' of Adam Smith in the marketplace of the eighteenth century may have been appropriate to medicine at that time.[4] It is much less so today. Indeed, it is only the asymmetry of information between patient and doctor that has, to date, allowed the medical profession to continue to act as if the individualistic ethics of virtue and responsibility were enough.

The fundamental issue here would seem to relate to the justified boundaries of medical power; that is, what are the property rights of doctors and what ought they to be? These are the questions that need to be answered.

The primary reason why medicine needs to reassess its medical ethics is not with respect to individual autonomy or dignity, nor partnership with the individual patient nor justice. Rather, the key issue is that in aggregate, as societies, we have lost the right to determine the objectives and priorities for 'our' health care systems. The primacy of the freedom of the individual – particularly the individual doctor but also the individual patient – in health care has thwarted efforts at genuine social choice in health care. No government has been prepared to take on the medical profession in the sense in which it matters; that is, to expose certain features (but by no means all) of their defence of current medical ethics and particularly clinical freedom as, in part, the usurping of democratic power in the name of doing good for the individual patient. In this, the individual patient has inevitably been willing to play along since it is in their interest (selfishly) to do so.

In raising these issues, my point is a simple one: there *is* a problem in medicine. The answer is not for the medical profession necessarily to adopt different values, although that might help. It is for society in aggregate to be better able to control and influence the objectives, directions and priorities of health care than it currently is and thereby exercise greater control and influence over the medical profession much more than it currently does.

As a member of society and as a potential patient, I have four fundamental interests in health care: (1) having good health care available to me; (2) having it available to everyone else in this society and with positive discrimination towards those disadvantaged as defined by the society; (3) ensuring that somebody, somewhere, keeps some check on the supply side of health care, since as an individual I cannot; and (4) insisting that the share of the nation's resources going on health care is reasonable, given all the other desirable things in my life. As a society, can we not recognise that a lot of the potential for attaining these goals rests in our own collective hands?

The purchaser–provider split or the internal market reforms of the UK National Health Service, the New Zealand health service and others in the context of some of the points made here on ethics and the role of societies in influencing health care objectives and priorities may be seen as backward steps. Whatever their other merits, their emphasis on the individual, and the ideas of freedom of choice and the virtues of choice were at best overstated and at worst misplaced.

There is a model of health care that emphasises the power of the market in the pursuit of efficiency. Whatever one's interpretation of the success of that model, there is no doubt that its roots lie in the ideas of the private market and the efficiency with which private markets act. Private markets can promote efficiency, but they require that several assumptions are fulfilled before this efficiency goal can be achieved. Not least among these is the need to have well-informed consumers. That is not the case in health care.[5] This is not to argue that consumer preferences are always inappropriate in health care, but there has to be some concern about the extent to which there are many occasions when the patient and the potential patient are well placed to exercise rational preferences. There are arguments for trying to get doctors to provide attractive waiting rooms, to be nice to their patients, and to take account of the time costs to patients of waiting in their surgeries. Provided that patients want and demand – i.e. are willing to pay (and sufficiently) for – such 'process' considerations, then there are good arguments for providing these features efficiently in health care.

But it is pertinent to ask whether such mechanisms can work with the delivery of health. Can we as patients recognise a good doctor? Indeed, can we distinguish a good doctor from a nice doctor?

The push for individualism and 'consumerism' that lies behind the internal market looks very much like a mistaken view of how to create efficiency in health care.

A more fundamental and general question can be asked. Do patients in principle want more freedom of choice? While the answer may be yes, there is a need to address this question rather than simply assume that more patient choice is itself a good thing. The Danes introduced the idea of patients in the public sector being able to choose their hospital. Very few have chosen to exercise that choice. I am not arguing that freedom of choice is of no value in health care. What I am suggesting is that this market-driven idea needs to be tested rather than assumed. If there is evidence that patients want more choice, then let the evidence state clearly in what contexts this is the case rather than adopt what too often appears to be an ideological blanket approach to such freedom of choice. Further, the fact that it is wanted does not mean that it should be supplied. The relationship between wants and demands applies here as well, as does the issue of the need to weigh up the costs and benefits of this intervention just as with any other proposed policy initiative.

These issues also involve certain ethical considerations about the social choices involved in health care. They are difficult ones to disentangle. There are few absolute rights and wrongs here, but there are possibilities for better and worse solutions. What is needed is not dogma but a genuine attempt to find out two things (which I do not think would prove so difficult): what do patients want from their doctors? And what do citizens want from their health services? Perhaps such an exercise would reveal that patients and citizens do want more freedom of choice, and in that respect I would then be proved wrong. More importantly than whether I am right or wrong, however, is that the question be put rather than the answer assumed.

7.3 The relevance of utilitarianism

In his classic text on medical ethics, Veatch examines a hypothetical island where pursuit of the concept of utilitarianism (which is clearly one way of defining the common good, and one frequently favoured by economists in cost–benefit analyses) appeared to create certain problems.[6] Given the task of identifying the best health care programme (i.e. the one that provided the greatest net benefit to the island), the planners discovered that the best buy 'would simultaneously reduce mortality rates, morbidity rates, infant mortality and other indicators of health problems ... and it would not be ... expensive ... or difficult to administer'.

However, this particular programme 'would require social scientists to identify the 1 per cent of the population that was chronically ill with incurable illness, possessing insufficient intelligence to follow a medical regimen and receiving expensive medical care. Excluding this population, which would be banned from receiving any further health care, a universal health maintenance system would be established for the island.'

The issue was then: should the island's government implement the programme? It is a thought-provoking and useful example, but I find it difficult to accept Veatch's statement that in such situations 'we are trapped between the ultra-individualism of the Hippocratic medical ethic and the social indiscrimination of utilitarians'.

Let us simplify his example. There is available on the island a very limited quantity of drug X. This has two unique properties: it can alleviate the pain of a group of 50 patients or it can save the lives of another group of 100 patients. Without it, the first group will exist in pain rather than without pain; the second group will die rather than live.

Set in these terms, not to relieve the pain of the first group may well be the best bet in terms of the net benefit to society at large. However, it need not be. If it is a caring society, then it is quite possible that the greatest net benefit will be provided by a programme that reduces the pain a little for the 50 at the expense of one death among the 100 who might have been saved. Indeed, this could be one explanation for resorting to the rule utility that Veatch suggests: 'The interests of society could be allowed to surface only in the formulation of principles or rules that would produce the greatest good in the long run'.[7]

That, however, seems not to be quite the point. Rather, it may be that what Veatch includes in his definition of utility is inadequate. While not explicit about this, it appears that he includes only the outcome utility in terms of health status changes. However, as mentioned briefly in the previous section, and as we will discuss in more detail in Chapter 9, the notion of process utility may also be relevant. If this is the case, then in addition to each individual islander's valuations of their own health status, we may have to add to the calculus:

- The valuation of each islander of the health status of all other islanders (which might in many cases be zero but in at least some would be positive); in other words, a measure of caring for others.
- The valuation of the islanders of the health care institution; that is, their valuations of health care may not be independent of the process involved in obtaining health care.

Build these in and utilitarianism seems to take on a new lease of life. For example, at one point Veatch argues that 'One of the problems of the utilitarian ethical principle is that, at least hypothetically, it seems to justify too much. It would have justified the Nazi experiments if only the Nazis had been clever enough to devise experiments that really produced benefit on balance.'[8] This is a most peculiar comment. Given the enormous cost in all sorts of dimensions and the lack or extremely limited benefit of the experiments the Nazis did conduct, it certainly doesn't seem likely that 'the utilitarian ethical principle' could be used to justify them at all. If they 'had been clever enough to devise experiments that really produced benefit on balance', then presumably the atrocities would not have occurred. There is some confused thinking here on Veatch's part. Certainly, for my part, I can only wish in this particular context that the Nazis had been utilitarians able with perfect foresight to weigh up the costs and benefits of their actions.

Other criticisms of utilitarianism arise from those who believe that it plays down the issue of individual autonomy and the concept of duty.

The difficulties here in the context of health care are essentially two. First, and as was discussed in detail in Chapters 3 and 5, the extent to which the individual is capable of reflection and judgement and has 'the capacity for choice', in the context of their choices for their health care, is limited. It is not even limited uniformly, being greater in primary care than in acute hospital care. Second, even if the individual does have the capacity or is given the capacity (and that is unlikely to be a costless exercise), it may well be that they simply do not want to do the choosing.

More recently, as a result of some of the difficulties here with some aspects of both medical ethics as is and utilitarianism in health care, I have been taken with some of the ideas of communitarianism, which shift the emphasis away from the values of the individual qua individual to the values of the community and the values on the community.

7.4 Communitarianism

Communitarians, such as Avineri and de-Shalit, argue:

> the premises of individualism such as the rational individual who chooses freely are wrong or false, and that the only way to understand human behaviour is to refer to individuals in their social, cultural, and historical contexts ... that the premises of individualism give rise to morally unsatisfactory consequences. Among them are the impossibility of achieving a genuine community, the neglect of some ideas of the good life that should be sustained by the state or others that should be dismissed, or – as some communitarians argue – an unjust

distribution of goods. In other words, the community is a good that people should seek for several reasons and should not be dismissed.'[9]

How can communitarianism be interpreted within the context of health care? One possibility is that considered by Margolis in Chapter 10. Individuals in society may be prepared to act (and acting has utility in its own right) to create a situation in which everyone – including themselves – has equal access to health care when in need. This is Margolis' 'participation utility' from which he developed his 'fair shares' model.

It is a short step from this to the idea that, with health services, individuals in a society may be prepared to pay to make available services for the population as a whole. Individuals get utility from the process of giving, which is additional to the utility from the knowledge that everyone has equal access.

The fact that the extent to which individuals in different societies may be prepared to do their fair share for that society seems to vary across different countries and cultures would lend support to the communitarian basis of such attitudes. Some communities, such as in the USA, seem to be more individualistic than others (e.g. Scandinavian countries). Even within individual countries there can be differences in the strength of community identity, such as between the Maori and non-Maori cultures in New Zealand. Individuals are not just individuals qua individuals; they are also members of some society, and such membership, to some extent at least, shapes their attitudes both as selfish individuals and as citizens.

The point, however, is that this is an element of communitarianism that does involve individual values, but they are individuals' values based on a clear recognition of the fact that individuals are members of a community and value being members of a community and as a result want that community to be a community in which they are happy to live. It is a part of the communitarian question.

Clearly, there will be occasions where different philosophies will come into conflict. What is essential is that medical ethics in practice should accept more than it currently does that there may be a role for utilitarianism in health care valuation and, consequently, for the ethics of the common good. At the same time, those including many economists may want to think of how better to express their concerns for the incorporation of the values of the community. Communitarianism may be the way forward here.

7.5 Conclusion

This chapter has attempted to highlight the source of the friction between economics and medicine: essentially, social versus individualistic ethical bases coming into conflict. There may be some people who would argue that making this conflict explicit is a mistake and that it is better to accept that doctors will pursue (legitimately so) clinical ends and that it has to be (legitimately) left to others to resolve the social and economic issues. In a sense I agree – if it were happening in that way. But it is by no means clear that it is.

This takes us back to the agency relationship as discussed in Chapter 6. There it was suggested that the doctor–patient relationship could be seen in the context of the doctor acting on behalf of the poorly informed patient. That would seem to be what much of medicine is about. I have no complaint with that. What would seem inappropriate is for the individual doctor to be in a position to affect the priorities for health care in the sense of the values of doctors being used in determining or influencing the allocation of resources between, for example, the old and the young, psychiatric care and maternity care, etc.

It is to be hoped and expected that a major part of the doctor's concern will be for the patient and not for themselves. But there have to be occasions when a conflict will arise at the level of doctor/patient or doctor (patient interest)/doctor (self-interest). An understanding of the motives involved and their strengths would seem to provide a focus for trying to ensure that the patient's manifest preferences do as often as possible and as far as possible end up as their true preferences. And the best way to achieve that is to make the terms of this conflict explicit.

There are clear issues of power here. There has to be concern on the part of the individual patient that no matter the extent to which the doctor operates out of patient interest, there remains the need for reassurance that this will always be the case and that the risk of exploitation by the informed supplier is minimised, as discussed previously in the context of the agency relationship in Chapter 6.

It would seem likely, however, that the risk of exploitation and the extent to which any level of such risk is seen as problematical will vary from country to country or perhaps from health care system to health care system. It can also be argued readily that attitudes to individuality are not constant over time.

Communitarianism may be a useful adjunct to our thinking in how to build health services as social institutions. (For a fuller account, see Mooney.[10]) There again, some societies are further down that road than others. There is unlikely to be a universally common or correct answer on how best to build ethical health care services.

Questions

1. What is it that both ethics and economics are about?
2. What are the principal theories of ethics?
3. Why are there medical ethical codes?
4. Do patients want freedom of choice?

5. What are the key features of utilitarianism?
6. What is communitarianism? How most importantly does it differ from utilitarianism?

Notes

1. J.C. Harsanyi, 'Morality and the theory of rational behaviour', in *Utilitarianism and Beyond*, eds. A. Sen and B. Williams (Cambridge University Press: Cambridge, 1982), p 55.
2. A. Sen and B. Williams, 'Introduction', in *Utilitarianism and Beyond*, eds A. Sen and B. Williams (Cambridge University Press: Cambridge, 1982), p 10.
3. A. Sen, *Inequality Re-examined* (Clarendon Press: Oxford, 1992).
4. A. Smith, *Wealth of Nations* (The Grand Colosseum Warehouse: Glasgow, 1869; first published 1776).
5. T. Rice, *The Economics of Health Reconsidered* (Health Administration Press: Chicago, 2002).
6. R.M. Veatch, *A Textbook of Medical Ethics* (Yale University Press: New Haven, 1981).
7. Ibid., p 175.
8. Ibid., p 174.
9. S. Avineri and A. de-Shalit, *Communitarianism and Individualism* (Oxford University Press: Oxford, 1992).
10. G. Mooney, 'Communitariansim and health economics', in *The Social Economics of Health Care*, ed. J.B. Davis (Routledge: London, 2001).

eight

Just health care: only medicine?

Mirror, mirror on the wall,
What is the fairest of them all?

8.1 Introduction

Whatever the financing mechanism, the question of justice and equity in health care seems important. Whatever else people dispute in health service policy, there is general agreement that fairness should be a part of health care. The weight that should be attached to the questions of what fairness is, or should be, is much less than immediately apparent.

What is discussed in this chapter initially is the uncertainty surrounding equity in health care. I do not argue that one definition is uniquely correct but instead point to the need for clarity in setting the goals of equity. Thereafter, some of the practical difficulties involved in pursuing equity are debated before highlighting some of the implications, particularly for other objectives such as efficiency, in choosing one equity objective rather than another. Finally, the chapter returns to issues of ethics, but specifically those related to equity. What emerges is that ethics and equity are interdependent, as are ethics and efficiency and, in turn, equity and efficiency. Perhaps that is inevitable. The explicit recognition of this, however, seems far from inevitable, particularly among the medical profession. There would appear to be a case for trying to change that.

8.2 What is equity?

In an attempt to highlight the definitional problems, it is worth listing a few possible definitions. These might be equality of:

- expenditure per capita
- inputs per capita
- inputs for equal need
- access for equal need
- utilisation for equal need
- marginal met need
- health.

There are practical problems in attempting to implement most of these notions of equity. Before discussing that issue, however, it is relevant to explain some of these definitions. The distinction between expenditure per capita and inputs per capita is simply that, as between two different areas of a country, prices of the relevant manpower, goods and services that comprise the inputs into health care may differ. As a result, a fixed level of expenditure may buy more inputs in one location than in another.

The distinction between access and utilisation is that the former is wholly a supply-side phenomenon and the latter is a function of both supply and demand (or need). In other words, equal access means that two (or more) individuals face the same costs to themselves of using the health care facility (e.g. it might be that they live the same distance from the facility, although this 'resource cost' definition is only one of two possibilities – see below). Whether they use it equally will be dependent on their valuation of that use; in other words, their demand for health and health care. Various aspects of this can be shown diagrammatically for visits to a general practitioner. From Figure 8.1, we can see that, if two individuals face equal costs of access and have equal demands for health care, utilisation of health care will also be the same. If they have different demands but equal access (Figure 8.2), or different access but equal demands (Figure 8.3), they will have different utilisation. If they have both different access and different demand, it is likely but not necessarily the case that their utilisation will differ (Figure 8.4). (Thus, in Figure 8.4, if the marginal cost curve for B had been a little higher, V(A) and V(B) would have been the same.)

These distinctions seem simple enough, and yet there is considerable confusion concerning these matters. There is no need for this, however.

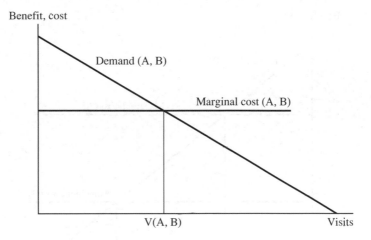

Figure 8.1 Equal access, equal demand

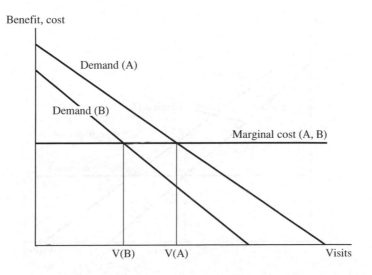

Figure 8.2 Equal access, different demand

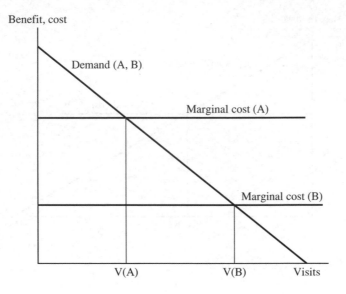

Figure 8.3 Equal demand, different access

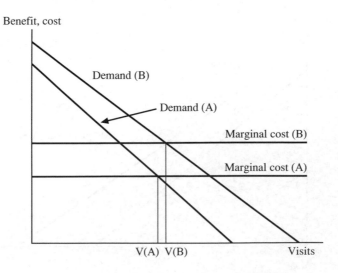

Figure 8.4 Different demand, different access

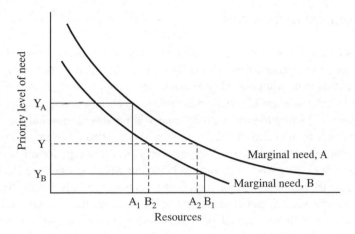

Figure 8.5 Marginal met need

Equality of marginal met need may warrant a little more explanation. It is based on the cost–benefit approach and was developed initially by Steele.[1] *Ceteris paribus*, a rational health authority operating under a budget constraint will allocate its scarce resources to those activities for which the ratios of benefits to costs are highest. It will continue to do this until it has used up its total allocation or expenditure. It will therefore want to establish ranking of needs to be met, the ranking being based on the size of the benefit/cost ratio involved in tackling different needs.

Adopting this process does not necessarily mean that something like heart transplants or kidney dialysis would be ranked highly. While success in these areas certainly would bring with it high benefits, it also brings high costs, and success may be far from certain. Consequently, it could be that high ranking will be associated with relatively low-benefit programmes if they happen to be low cost as well.

Diagrammatically, if we were concerned with equity regionally in a country, the picture we would get for equating marginal met need in two different regions would be as in Figure 8.5.

Let us assume that initially the resources available are A_1 in region A and B_1 in region B. The needs just met are Y_A in A and Y_B in B. To equate marginal met need requires a redistribution of the total resources available ($A_1 + B_1$) until both regions are meeting the same marginal need. This occurs at A_2 and B_2 (note that $A_2 + B_2$ must equal $A_1 + B_1$) when the marginal met need is the same (i.e. Y).

8.3 Practical difficulties

Problems in practice will vary depending on what definition is chosen. However, they all relate to measurement, primarily of need but also of the groups across which we want to be equitable. (For example, there are problems in defining social classes.) In order to highlight these difficulties and at the same time to discuss the practicalities of getting to grips with the equity issue, this section outlines the way in which resource allocation issues for equity are handled conventionally. This is based on the Resource Allocation Working Party (RAWP)-type formulae that have been used across the globe, with various bells and whistles, since the RAWP first promulgated the approach over a quarter of a century ago in England.[2] In various guises and with various twists and turns, and at various times in the intervening period, this approach has been adopted in a number of countries and locations (see, for example, NSW Health Department,[3] BC Ministry of Health,[4] and Scottish Executive[5]). Later in this chapter an alternative, preferred way is presented.

Despite the attempt by the WHO to impose a common objective on all countries, the emphasis placed on the objective of equity in health care and how it is defined inevitably varies from one country to another.[6] Many of the problems in this area are nonetheless common. Consequently, while the example here is drawn from work that originated in the UK, it has much wider relevance. The RAWP Formula set the scene for a series of resource-allocation formulae in many countries. Indeed, the publication in 1976 of the formula sparked off an international industry in regional resource-allocation formulae. There have been a number of different versions, but the fundamentals remain.

The original RAWP was the official response of the UK government to the question of whether it is fair or equitable for an individual to be penalised in their access to health care simply because of what part of the country they happen to live in. Or again, is there any reason why one region of the country should receive more per capita by way of resources than another region?

With regard to the relevant organisational features of the NHS, all that is necessary to know is that:

- The NHS is funded very largely through central government taxes and is mainly zero money priced at the point of consumption.
- The government has to divide the total budget available between the various regional health authorities, who have responsibility for administering the services in each region.
- RAWP was about how to divide that cake up equitably.

The methods used before RAWP to distribute financial resources from the centre to the regions were largely supply-oriented. In other words, they were influenced heavily by what facilities happened to exist and therefore happened to be taken over by the NHS when it was established in 1948.

The stated objective of RAWP was couched in terms of equal opportunity of access for those at equal risk. It should also be stressed that RAWP was concerned with need, not supply or demand. Consequently, the approach adopted was aimed at measuring relative need for health care in different regions and then allocating expenditures pro rata with these estimates of relative needs.

The factors deemed relevant to estimates of relative need were as follows:

- *Size of population*: on the simple basis that health care is for people. In passing, it is worth noting that population size is always likely to prove the biggest factor in determining relative need for health care for different groups in society.
- *Composition*: the elderly and the young tend to have greater need for health care than those in the middle age range. Also, women and men have different health needs. Consequently, the age/sex composition of the population will affect estimates of relative need.
- *Morbidity*: the more sick a population is, *ceteris paribus*, the greater is its need for health care.
- *Cost*: some conditions may prove more expensive to treat than others, so the nature of morbidity may be relevant. Again, the cost of providing facilities may vary between regions; for example, salary levels for the same grades of staff may vary, or economies of scale may not be capable of being reaped as readily in sparsely populated, rural areas as in dense, urban areas.
- *Patient cross-boundary flows*: there may be patient flows into or out of various regions.
- *Medical education*: this is not spread equally across the different regions, and some allowance will need to be made for this.
- *Capital investment*: while capital allocations for new building and so on will be influenced by the factors listed above, it may also be necessary to adjust for not only quantitative differences in capital stock but also differences in qualitative factors such as age.

One of the difficulties in pursuing a formula incorporating all these factors in estimating relative regional needs is that the needs for all these services cannot be assumed to be influenced to the same extent by them. Another problem is that the information required to estimate the needs is not always available, at least not in an ideal form.

To overcome the first problem, services can be disaggregated into different categories (e.g. inpatient non-psychiatric, inpatient pyschiatric, community services, etc.), with the overall spend on each category set out. Whatever the relevant factors in estimating sickness need for each particular service, they can be applied at, say, a regional level to establish what proportion that region has of total sickness need for illnesses falling into that category. That can then provide the estimate of the proportion of the total spend in that category of services (e.g. non-psychiatric inpatient services), which then gets allocated to that region. The total budget for that region is then an aggregation of the spends calculated for each set of services.

What does this mean in practice? First, the population size is estimated – say, five million people; then it must be determined whether the people in that area tend to be rather old and, allowing for their age, whether they are rather more sick (this is the standardised mortality ratio (SMR), of which more below) than the average nationally: in which case, they should get an extra allowance in funding (at the expense of a younger, healthier region). The extent of this increase in this context should be determined by national bed-utilisation rates for different conditions. If age and sickness mean that this region's health needs are ten per cent above the average, then the 'notional' population becomes not five million but 5.5 million. Thus, assuming a total population of 50 million, the proportion of the budget available for non-psychiatric inpatient services going to this region should be not ten per cent (i.e. five in 50 million) but 11 per cent (i.e. 5.5 in 50 million). If the overall spend on non-psychiatric inpatients is, say, 60 per cent of the total, then 11% of 60 per cent of the total budget should be allocated to this region for these services (i.e. 6.6%). To this would then be added the allocation for the other services. Cross-boundary flow and teaching adjustments would follow on.

While there is a great deal of logic to this approach, there are weaknesses in it. These are basically as follows:

- It assumes that relative total need is a meaningful concept (doubtful, given the discussion in Chapter 6).
- It assumes that relative total need can be measured sufficiently accurately by relatively few factors.
- The measurement of relative morbidity used is suspect (again, readers will be ready to understand the difficulties here given the discussion on output measurement in Chapter 4).

On the third problem, the measure of morbidity used is usually the SMR. This statistic compares the number of deaths actually occurring in a region with those that would be expected if the national mortality ratios by age and sex were applicable to the population of that region. The reason for using this statistic as a measure of relative morbidity is simply that there are seldom any good and reliable measures of relative morbidity available.

The extent to which RAWP-type formulae have been used and have been subject to debate about their fairness in various countries makes them particularly interesting examples of attempts to put health care equity into a mathematical formula. It has, in various guises and with various shifts in emphasis, survived very well. It is argued, however, that there are more fundamental flaws in this approach that have been revealed only recently.

8.4 An alternative approach based on 'capacity to benefit'[7]

This section discusses an alternative process for allocating resources across different geographical areas. It is based on the simple idea that resources should be allocated to provide as much good as possible. This emphasis on the nature of the good is, in itself, somewhat novel. As indicated in Chapter 4, it is often assumed that health services are about maximising health, and concerns tend to be restricted to this (largely efficiency) question. When resource-allocation formulae do address equity, as indicated above, they tend to draw heavily on the notion of 'health need' or 'sickness need', the idea being that the greater this is – essentially the greater the health problems – the more money should be allocated. At first sight, it might appear logical to argue that the size of the problem should determine the amount of resources to be allocated to trying to fix the problem. The 'capacity to benefit' (CTB) approach outlined here challenges this. Once the notion of trying to do good is introduced, then what dominates in the resource-allocation question is not the size of the problem but rather how much good can be done with whatever resources are available.

It is also the case that with respect to the use of SMRs, where populations have been standardised for age, then because older people tend to use more resources than younger people, other things being equal, if one population is older than another, that population will get more resources. That seems logical, provided that the object is set in terms of allocating according to need in terms of sickness. Yet where a population is so sick that it never, on average, gets old (as is the case, for example, with some Aboriginal populations), then the use of SMRs instead of discriminating in favour of the disadvantaged will in fact penalise them for dying young!

While at first sight this appears most strange, the explanation is simple. The sickness-based needs approach – what has been described above as a RAWP-type formula – allocates according to the size of the problem as it is. It does not look at the issue of trying to ameliorate the problem or of assessing what the impact might be in terms of where populations end up rather than where they start, in other words in terms of the value added by the resources. This alternative approach is about looking to see what capacity there is to change things as well as being concerned with equity. This is why it is called *the capacity to benefit approach.*

In this new approach developed by the author and Shane Houston[8], it is argued that account should be taken of the preferences of those patients and citizens who are to benefit from the resources allocated. For example, this was done in Western Australia for the Aboriginal population. What is then crucial in this approach is to ensure that there is an appropriate conceptual base (that of capacity to benefit) but that also makes due allowance for the preferences of the people who will be affected directly by the resources allocated.

There are four components to the approach used in Western Australia. These have to be brought together in such a way as to reflect as well as possible whatever good is to be achieved with the resources available.

First, there is an assessment of the benefit that additional resources might provide, i.e. *CTB*. There is then a need to weight this to reflect the fact that society might want to give a higher weight to benefits to disadvantaged people. This is the concern of *vertical equity*, which attempts to provide some notion of positive discrimination.

The third component embraces the fact that communities are not developed equally well in terms of their infrastructures to allow them to have the capacity to benefit from additional resources for, say, an eye programme. Because of the multifaceted nature of this phenomenon, it has been called *management, economic, social and human* (MESH) *infrastructure*.

The fourth component concerns reducing inequities in terms of access to services whether this be for reasons of distance or culture. To deal with *geographical remoteness* and *cultural access barriers* would require additional resources.

In operationalising the approach, there is a need to respect informed local preferences to determine the nature of the good that the relevant resources are aimed at achieving. The driving force is equity, with emphasis on CTB, but allowing added weight to the relatively disadvantaged, providing funds to build up infrastructure that is currently lacking (such as management and leadership skills) and also compensating those areas where there are added barriers to use of services as a result of distance or other access problems.

Too often in the past it seems that consideration of the availability of data has been the driving force in devising such resource allocation formulae and hence the popularity of RAWP-type formulae. There are problems in applying this CTB type of approach, mostly with respect to data availability. Conceptually, however, the CTB approach seems superior on all other counts.

8.5 How should equity be defined?

There is no uniquely correct way of defining equity. It is dependent on a value judgement both about equity per se and about the relative weight to be attached to it vis-à-vis other objectives of any health care system. One aspect of this that requires close examination is the potential trade-off between equity and efficiency.

By way of example, let us assume that the definition of equity we are using is 'equality of access for equal need' (see page 74). Assume, too, that the country we are considering is composed of one large island with a population of 490,000 and five small islands, each with a population of 2000. There is a major teaching hospital on the main island, but the small islands are served solely by local general practitioners. In such circumstances, whatever the overall level of spending on health care, it seems inevitable that equal access to high-quality inpatient hospital care can be bought only at a high price. And if we assume that the budget is fixed, then that price must be in terms of health care facilities and, we can assume, health. Consequently, there can be a trade-off between equity and efficiency. Thus, maximising health may not be achievable from a given budget where another objective relates to equity.

This trade-off, however, will not always be present. Where the issue is one of dealing equally with equals (horizontal equity), then equity and efficiency will tend to move together. However, in vertical equity – the unequal but equitable treatment of unequals – there is likely to be a conflict with efficiency. For example, in the context of prevention, it may be that reducing risks a little for the majority of the population will save fewer lives than concentrating the same resources on the few people who are at high risk. An added difficulty with vertical equity is determining the degree of inequality that exists and deciding the extent to which that justifies or merits treatment inequalities. Clearly, the problems of output measurement, discussed in detail in Chapter 4, arise here with a vengeance.

Broadly, as we move through the definitions of equity listed earlier in this chapter, it will tend to be the case that the trade-off with efficiency will increase (although note that equality of marginal met need does not fit this trend.) If, for example, given all the other influences on health outside the health service, the choice of the definition of equity should be equality of health, presumably age-standardised, in so far as this is at all feasible, it could only be at a very low level of health. In other words, equal health would mean equally bad health.

Consequently, in any decision on what the equity goal is to be, it is important to attempt to assess the impact of that choice on other health service goals. It is not enough to want to pursue an efficient, equitable health care policy. Questions have to be posed about *how* efficient and *how* equitable.

There is a lot of appeal, in principle at least, in the CTB approach (which builds on the marginal met need idea of Steele[9] and Culyer's capacity to benefit notion of need.[10] It avoids the problems thrown up by RAWP-type formulae of attempting to measure relative total need in different regions and concentrates firmly on trying to maximise the good. It allows local communities to determine what they mean by 'good' but still takes care of equity by, first, weighting benefits according to degrees of disadvantage and, second, permitting a funding allowance to build up community capabilities where these may be deficient. On the basis of various surveys of colleagues, students, health service decision-makers and the public, in practice it appears that, faced with the choice between the seven definitions presented above, most opt for equal access for equal need. This definition can be left like that, or it can be made more complex or sophisticated. See, for example, the Perth Citizens' Jury definition later in this chapter.[11]

There is no uniquely correct answer to the question, 'what is equity in health care?' Equality of utilisation is, in my view, too elitist. I cannot accept the notion of compulsory health care: 'You will use the health service just like the sensible middle classes.' Equality of health is simply too expensive in terms of sacrifices to health and other good things in this life.

8.6 Equity and ethics

There are many who would argue that equity in health care is a matter of ethics, an issue already touched on in Chapter 7.

Veatch, in his classic work on medical ethics, discusses four theories of justice.[12] The first of these – entitlement theory – suggests that we are all entitled to what we have, provided we have acquired it justly. The well-to-do have no obligation to help the less-well-to-do; the distribution of entitlements is essentially a matter of luck, and the lucky have no duty to look after the unfortunates. It is, in effect, an amoral theory of justice. However, as soon as one concedes that some existing distribution of resources is less than fair – surely especially true of the distribution of health – the theory would seem to fall apart.

Utilitarianism, Veatch's second theory of justice, has already been discussed in detail in Chapter 7. He states that the approach of 'serving the greatest good for the greatest number ... is a favourite strategy of health planners and economists'. But utilitarianism is not really a theory of justice. Indeed, one of the criticisms made of it is that it is devoid of any ethics of justice. It is essentially about efficiency, not equity.

Veatch then looks at the maximin theory, best exemplified in Rawls' theory of justice,[13] and that relates very much to the idea that there is some duty or simply wish that the worst off be given high priority. If people operating behind a veil of ignorance such that they do not know their position in society were asked what sort of society they wished for, Rawls suggests they would opt for one of maximising benefit to the least well off. Such a proposal says nothing about the costs to the rest of society in pursuing such a policy – a rather important consideration in a world not hiding behind a veil of ignorance.

Veatch's fourth theory of justice is the theory of egality, essentially the 'equality of net welfare for individuals'. For this, in the context of health care, equality of health would be the goal.

What is important for our discussion is to note that these ethical overtones are present in much of this discussion, at least in two of these theories – maximin and egalitarianism. It is studiously omitted from the entitlement theory and played down and perhaps even missing from the utilitarian theory. More discussion of these issues in Chapter 9 will, I think, reveal that there are considerable advantages in accepting what is essentially a utilitarian non-ethical view of justice and one that avoids the problems of imposing an unwanted (and hence one bearing negative utility) code of justice on the society concerned.

But what of equity in the context of the medical profession? Is there a justice that they do or should subscribe to? This would seem to be the case in health care systems that attempt to treat patients according to need rather than demand, in other words where the basis of treatment is related to the sickness of the patients or their capacity to benefit rather than the patients' willingness and ability to pay. Where the ability of patients to pay enters into the equation, then issues of inequity arise. It may be argued that this is a systems issue and not one that is for medical doctors to be concerned about, i.e. the doctors act ethically by treating equally or fairly all those who present to them, and it is beyond their domain of influence as individual doctors to be concerned about those who do not present. That seems fair enough, but there may also be ethical issues for the individual doctor in deciding in what system or where in the system to practise. Are there, for example, ethical choices for doctors that have a bearing on equity in choosing where to practise in the public or private or both sectors, or rural or remote areas, or poor or rich areas? Is it even fair to suggest that these choices are ethical ones for doctors, or should incentives within the system be devised to make them more ethical choices for the system and less so for individual doctors? These are thorny questions that I will leave up in the air.

What is clear, however, is that there is no ethical duty on doctors with respect to how their actions affect resource deployment in health care to act efficiently or equitably. Doctors (except, perhaps, those in public health) are not trained to act efficiently or equitably vis-à-vis resource allocation. They are not well placed to know the costs of their actions. It might even be argued that it would be unethical for them to take account of costs in their decision-making. What does become problematical, however, is that, if clinicians are to divorce themselves in their clinical decision-making from the ethics of resource allocation, then they cannot be involved outside the clinical arena in such debate.

There are, I believe, some simple guidelines here that revolve around opportunity costs. I do not think that anyone would dispute that, in the clinical arena, it is for the clinical doctor to decide how best to use their time. The doctor is the best person to decide to spend a few extra minutes with patient A rather than patient B. That argument might be extended to clinical resource allocation more generally, although that would depend on how budgets are allocated and constrained. In other words, within the clinical arena the doctor is best placed to judge not only what benefit is obtained by these few minutes with patient A but also the opportunity cost in not spending these same few minutes with patient B. The doctor seems less well placed to judge whether their time in surgery is more valuable than another doctor's time in medicine, or a community nurse's time visiting an elderly person, or the time of a teacher or an army captain or a cinematographer. The judgements at this level of opportunity cost are no longer clinical. They are hospital-wide or health-service-wide or public-service-wide or social. Opportunity cost is very precise in the sense that it always means the benefit foregone in the best alternative use of resources. This best, however, varies depending on what resource or budget constraint operates. As that varies, so too does the relevant individual or group who can or should exercise that value judgement.

Two of the key features in this are the separation of advice from action and of the individual from the society. The two in fact ought to be linked. Those who are to advise on equity and efficiency ought to do so from a standpoint that is much wider than either the individual patient or indeed the individual practitioner and their patients. There has to be a strong case for those who proffer such advice being separated from the demands and prejudices of individual patient care.

Hence emerges the role of the community physician but, in a much wider and more important sense, also the role of the representatives of the society at large, no matter who they may be. Issues of equity and efficiency in health care are not the sole ethical province of the medical profession. Indeed, it can be argued that they are not the province of the medical profession outside of community medicine except as doers of society's will. In terms of equity and efficiency, clinicians need to be the advised, not the advisers.

These are vexed issues. Writing ethical codes is fraught with difficulty. Equity, efficiency and ethics in health care are not solely medical matters; indeed, in many instances in terms of relevant policy-making they are not medical matters at all.

Let me exemplify what I mean. If it were the case that the medical profession's values should determine priorities in health care, then would it be wrong to leave the individual members of the profession to make their case to the relevant administrative and political bodies and let resource allocation be based on the strength of the cases put forward? My answer is no, but with two provisos: first, that cases be made on a rational basis; and second, that cases be made at the same level of decibels. The people with the muscle are in the acute specialties – the top surgeons and physicians; the weak are in the Cinderella services for the elderly, the mentally ill and the handicapped. Left to the individualistic ethics of medicine, the acute sector will tend to win. In terms of justice and allocative efficiency – and therefore in terms of social ethics – it perhaps ought not to. So the fact that power is not distributed fairly within the medical profession makes the members of that august body even less well qualified for advising on justice and efficiency in resource allocation.

It is also the case that, left to the doctors and the medical associations, teaching hospitals will attract more resources than would be the case if these decisions were left to others in health care or indeed to society at large. In Perth, Australia, there is an excellent example of this, where an Aboriginal Medical Service (AMS) had to close a branch because of overspending, while the teaching hospitals overspent by over 100 times as much and were not subjected to any assessment of their financial management and got bailed out.

These are key issues for the fair and efficient management of health services. They are central to the ethical dilemmas facing health care policy-makers under all sorts of financing and organisational systems. We will return to them again in Chapter 11 after a sojourn into wider issues of equity and ethics; that is, the nature of health care systems and why these vary from country to country.

8.7 What's best?

A major question (so far unanswered in this chapter) with respect to equity is the one that Sen poses: what is in the evaluative space?[14] There is no agreed uniquely correct *definition* of equity in health care, nor is there agreement as to how important equity is as a health care objective. Given that equity is inevitably a value-laden, social and cultural phenomenon, it would be wrong to think that there could be such agreement. Even within an individual country, it is unlikely that there would be an agreed definition of or weight attached to equity, and certainly this is true as between, for example, non-Aboriginal and Aboriginal Australians.

There are, as discussed, a range of possibilities. The most common are equal health, equal access (for equal need) and equal use (for equal need). Within these, there are different interpretations (for example, both access and need can be construed in different ways). Donaldson and Gerard suggest that in the countries they examined the most common definition of equity is equal access for equal need.[15]

There are also different ways of conceiving of equity. For example, horizontal equity is about the equal treatment of equals, while vertical equity is about the unequal but equitable treatment of unequals. It is also possible to distinguish usefully between distributive justice and procedural justice, where the former is consequentialist and concerned only with outcomes and the latter with the fairness of processes or procedures.

I am loath to advocate any particular definition of equity. I believe this is a decision that should be made on an informed basis by the relevant community or society. To date, they are seldom if ever given the chance to do so. One example, that at least starts down this road, is the equity stance that Citizens' Juries, with membership selected randomly from the electoral roll, adopted at a meeting in Australia organised under the auspices of the WA Medical Council.[16] Their definition of equity may be summarised as follows:

> Equal access for equal need, where equality of access means that two or more groups face barriers of the same height and where the judgement of the heights is made by each group for their own group; where need is defined as capacity to benefit; and where nominally equal benefits may be weighted according to social preferences such that the benefits to more disadvantaged groups may have a higher weight attached to them than those to the better off.

This rather sophisticated and thoughtful definition allows for a number of features. First, the concept permits consideration of whatever the potential users perceive as barriers to use and the importance they attach to the various components of these barriers. Thus, cultural and racist barriers, if these are perceived to exist, can be included in the concept of access. Second, the definition avoids the somewhat sterile construct of need as amount of sickness, as discussed above. It concentrates instead on the scope for providing extra benefits to different groups (i.e. value added). Third, by weighting benefits differentially according to degrees of disadvantage, it endorses vertical equity.

The definition does not, however, address certain other problems that are worthy of note. First, it is implied that all groupings, social and cultural, will have the same perceptions or constructs of health or of health needs. This is a very common assumption or presumption in definitions of equity. It is, in fact, difficult to see how any of the three main definitions of equal health, equal access for equal need, and equal use for equal need can avoid incorporating a common construct of health or of health need. Yet even within the one country, the construct of health may not be the same for all, as is the case, for example, in Australia, where it is not the same for Aboriginal people as it is for non-Aboriginal Australians (see Houston[17]). Distributive justice in health care, however, and as indicated above, requires measured outcomes or consequences, involving health or health need. The implication of this is that it may not be possible, even if desirable, to work in practice with distributive justice. If there is no common outcome, in this instance a common construct of health, then making distributive justice operational is problematical.

This issue is worth stressing. No matter how equity in health care is defined, a notion of health is bound to be present, whether it be set in terms of health per se or health need. The difficulty then faced is that, since health is a culturally specific construct, any concept of equality built into a definition of equity that also involves health or need is likely to be faced with the problem of attempting to equalise disparate entities. How can we allocate health care resources equitably from a single budget when health is conceived differently by two or more cultures?

Second, if not all groupings have the same ability to 'manage to desire',[18] then this is likely to create problems in this definition. If the capacity to desire of two cultures is different (thus *inter alia* removing the prospects of using utility as a common measuring rod), how can we proceed? These vexed issues are addressed in more detail later.

Clearly that is an unsatisfactory note on which to end. Some of these problems will be greater in some countries than others. The problems are not insurmountable. What is needed in most countries is much more attention on equity in health care, much more debate about what it is, and greater resources being allocated to allow equity goals to be pursued.

Questions

1. How can equity in health care be defined?
2. How should it be defined?
3. What was RAWP?
4. How do sickness-based need and capacity-to-benefit need differ?
5. How do horizontal and vertical equity differ?
6. Are equity, efficiency and ethics in health care solely medical matters?
7. How might vertical equity be incorporated into a resource-allocation formula?

Notes

1. R. Steele, 'Marginal met need and geographical equity in health care', *Scottish Journal of Political Economy*, 28 (1981), pp 186–195.
2. Department of Health and Social Security, Resource Allocation Working Party report (Department of Health and Social Security: London, 1976).
3. NSW Health Department, 'Implementation of the economic statement for health', (NSW Health Department: Sydney, 1996).
4. BC Ministry of Health, 'Regional funding formula' (BC Ministry of Health: Vancouver, 1996).
5. Scottish Executive, *The Arbuthnott Formula* (Scottish Executive: Edinburgh, 2002).
6. World Health Organization, *The World Health Report* (WHO: Geneva, 2000).
7. G. Mooney and S. Houston, 'Weighted capacity to benefit and MESH infrastructure', SPHERe discussion paper (Curtin University: Perth, 2002).
8. Ibid.
9. Steele, op. cit.
10. A.J. Culyer, 'Need: the idea won't do – but we still need it', *Social Science and Medicine*, 40 (1995), pp 727–730.
11. Medical Council, 'What's fair in health care?' (Medical Council, Health Department of Western Australia: Perth, 2001).
12. R.M. Veatch, *A Theory of Medical Ethics* (Basic Books: New York, 1980).
13. J. Rawls, *A Theory of Justice* (Oxford University Press: Oxford, 1972).
14. A. Sen, 'Equality of what?', in *The Tanner Lectures on Human Values*, Vol. 1, ed. S.M. McMurrin (Cambridge University Press: Cambridge, 1980).
15. C. Donaldson and K. Gerard, *The Economics of Financing Health Care: The Visible Hand* (Macmillan: Basingstoke, 1993).
16. Medical Council, op. cit.
17. S. Houston, 'Aboriginal cultural security', (Health Department of Western Australia, Perth, 2001).
18. A. Sen, *Inequality Re-examined* (Clarendon Press, Oxford, 1992).

nine

Priority setting in health care

Doctors know the value of everything and the cost of nothing (to misquote Oscar Wilde).

9.1 Introduction

There is a sense in which priority setting is what economics is about. Economics is the science or the art of choice. Limited resources are to be allocated in such a way as to maximise benefits and at the same time ensure that health services are allocated in a way that is fair in the eyes of the society served. Given its importance, this chapter discusses the issues surrounding priority setting in some detail.

This chapter does three things. First, it discusses how economic analysis can be used to help to set priorities in health care. Second, it mounts a critique of QALY league tables. Third, it identifies some of the problems from an economic perspective in other approaches.

While writing this chapter, I was aware of the frustrations I have that economics is not accepted more in the field of priority setting. The merits of the economic approach to priority setting seem so obvious to me. Using economic analysis in an ideal fashion can be difficult, given in particular the demands on measuring techniques, especially of the benefits of health care, which are still being developed. There are also data deficiencies in all health care systems in the sense that, on both the costs and the benefits sides, the information does not exist in the form, detail and precision that is ideally wanted.

Yet a lot of these measurement and data problems are there whatever methods are used to address priorities; and frequently the methods adopted are deficient. Rational priorities in health care cannot be set without knowing about the costs and benefits of different patterns of intervention. It is thus not the approach of economics to priority setting that creates these problems. They exist. In so far as other approaches sidestep these problems, they cannot be genuinely useful methods of priority setting in getting us further down the road to more efficient and equitable health services.

This issue is important. Most of the criticisms that I hear regarding the economic approach to priority setting seem to centre largely on the practical problems of implementation. The concerns are almost exclusively with the data demands and the demands on measuring techniques that the economic approach makes.

As will be clear by this stage of the book, economics is first and foremost a way of thinking about resource allocation. In priority setting, this is especially true. The key message of this chapter is that unless the thinking underlying priority setting is 'right' – and there is scope for debate about precisely what 'right' means – then there is no possibility, except by luck, of getting priorities set in such a way that they will further the objectives of health care. It may well be the case in the foreseeable future that economic analysis in priority setting will not be implemented in any ideal fashion. However, an inadequate data and measuring set supporting the right thinking is more likely to get us to an approximation of where it is desirable to be than will better data and better measuring techniques where the thinking is wrong.

9.2 Priority setting using an explicit economics approach

The essence of priority setting from an economics perspective starts from the assumption that resources are scarce. This raises two considerations: first, the concept of opportunity cost is to the fore; second, the idea of meeting total need is simply not possible and indeed not worthy of contemplation. The starting point is therefore scarce resources.

This means getting an idea of how resources are currently being used, which is best done through programme budgeting. Thereafter, the question to be addressed is how best any changes in resource use can be made, be it through some redeployment of, reductions in, or increases in existing resources. This is the process normally referred to as marginal analysis. It is simple and involves considering whether a shift of resources of, say, Z from programme, project or procedure A to programme, project or procedure B will result in an increase in total benefits from the resources available. If it does, then the principle lying behind the approach suggests that the movement of resources should take place. The process is then repeated until no further shift of resources is worthwhile (in the sense of leading to a gain in total net benefit). Thus, the economic approach is a combination of programme budgeting and marginal analysis (PBMA), with the key concepts being opportunity cost and the margin. (For a useful survey on PBMA, see Mitton and Donaldson.[1])

I have sometimes suggested when teaching health economics that, if any of the participants falls asleep during my lecture and awakens conscious that I have asked a question but that it has gone unheard, then the best response is to mutter something about opportunity cost and the margin. This has something like a 50 per cent or higher chance of being at least partly right. In this particular case, opportunity cost and the margin say it all if the question concerns the key economic concepts in priority setting. It is worth emphasising this point, as we will see later that other methods used to set priorities often omit one or both of these concepts.

Programme budgeting is a simple mechanism for providing an information framework to assist the process of allowing resource use and outputs generated to be set alongside health service objectives and for helping to identify and begin the examination of relevant margins through marginal analysis. Programme budgeting is not evaluative in itself but creates a framework in which evaluation is facilitated and encouraged.

In any health authority, it will be possible to identify a series of broad programmes, for example by disease group – cancer, respiratory disease, etc.; by client group – the elderly, mentally ill, etc.; or perhaps by geographical location. There is a range of possibilities. However, the distinguishing feature of programmes is that they are output-oriented rather than input-oriented, as is the case with standard budgetary procedures. This is because, while the total spending on nurses (an input), for example, is an important piece of information in managing health services, the role of programme budgeting is to allow planning of health care and priority setting across different aspects of health care in ways that relate to the objectives of health care. It is this 'objectives' orientation that requires programme budgeting to be output-oriented. More simply, it might be said that the designation of programmes ought to be such that all programmes can have health care objectives associated with them, which is clearly the case for maternity care or cancer therapy. It is this output and objectives orientation that distinguishes programme budgeting from other forms of budgeting.

It is also potentially important that these programmes can be disaggregated into sub-programmes, such as, in the context of maternity care, antenatal care, the labour/birth period, and postnatal care. For each programme and eventually each sub-programme, the task is to set out what is being spent on each and also what is being achieved with each. For the latter, while the most accurate and appropriate indicator as possible of output should be used, in reality it will often be some readily available (and hence very often rather imprecise) measure that will be used, such as occupied bed days or discharges or consultations. It may also be useful to do this for more than the most recent year for which data are available, and go back to establish what trend there has been over the last few years. Here, much will depend on data availability and the precise purpose of the planning and priority setting exercise.

While there are various ways in which these tasks might be accomplished, it would seem sensible to establish a programme group or programme management group for each of the programmes. These might comprise professional staff working with the patients in the programme group – doctors, nurses, etc., managers for the programme, information and finance staff, and perhaps lay representatives. How such groups are set up will again depend on the local circumstances, but some grouping into programme management groups will certainly be needed to get the process working in practice.

Having set up programmes and sub-programmes and estimated the levels of expenditures on these and the outputs from them for at least one year and perhaps more, the scene is set – we have the information framework to begin to consider marginal shifts in resources. In practice, it might be that particular programmes can be analysed on the margin without actually setting out the programme budgets, as suggested above. However, it is my experience that the health service managers involved do not have a clear idea about what is contained within particular programmes, nor any real idea of the size of different parts of the total expenditures within programmes. As a result, they welcome the push that programme budgeting provides to specify the contents of programmes and to get a handle on the sizes of the expenditures involved in fairly broad terms in both programmes and sub-programmes.

It is also the case that the designation of programmes, and just as much sub-programmes, is a particularly important aspect of the process. This is because every division of the cake, be it between programmes or within programmes, constitutes a possible boundary across which resources may be moved. It is likely to be in the same terms that the margins will be defined when marginal analysis is undertaken.

Three questions can be asked:

- If there are no more resources available, can, say, £1 million be moved from programme X to programme Y and the overall total benefit be increased?
- If more resources are made available, on which programme or sub-programme are these additional resources best spent in the sense of creating most extra benefit?
- If expenditures are to be cut, where should the cut occur so that the impact in terms of loss of benefit is minimised?

The theory underlying this approach is simple. On the margin of each programme or sub-programme, for some fixed size of budget allocated across the whole set of programmes, the optimal allocation of the budget occurs where the ratio of marginal benefit to marginal cost is the same across all programmes or sub-programmes.

This is equivalent to saying that, if it is possible to move £Z from A to B and as a result increase the overall total benefit (i.e. the gain in B is greater than the loss of benefit in A), then this represents an improvement in efficiency and, as such, should be done. Such moves should continue until it is the case that no further movement of funds will result in still greater benefits being provided. When this stage is reached with respect to all programmes, i.e. it is not possible to provide still greater benefits unless more resources *in toto* are provided, that is the optimal situation with respect to efficiency.

With respect to the measurement of benefits, this might move in the direction of trying to establish a QALY league table or some health gain or benefit gain league table (see below). Certainly, any step in this direction will be useful, but it is as well to recognise that in the current state of the art any assessment of benefit will be less than precise. Of course, there is no way of removing totally the subjectivity involved in such choices – to trade off health gains for the elderly versus health gains for children has to be subjective. There may not, however, be very good information available even on the technical issue of the likely impact on health and other benefits of various ways of using the extra monies. This has to be accepted and overcome to the extent that available analytical resources or the existing literature on effectiveness will allow.

The same problems exist, of course, when there is a need to think about reductions in various programmes or sub-programmes. Again, there may be at best poor information about the benefit losses likely to occur in these circumstances.

It is also unlikely that there will be a lot of information readily available about the marginal costs of the various changes that might be considered as possibles for shifting resources. There are likely to be data about average costs, and while there will be a great temptation to use these the chances are very strong that the use of these average cost figures will lead to the costings being wrong. It is not that we can automatically assume that average costs will be different from marginal costs, but to assume that they will be different rather than assuming that they will be the same is a much better starting point.

Many costing studies would thus be needed, which in itself could be a very big exercise. To avoid this potentially long and time-consuming process, which could tie up the relatively few staff available for conducting analyses for the priority-setting exercises as a whole, this stage of the procedure is split into three. First, the programme management groups are asked to draw up wish lists but without at that stage having good data available on either benefits or costs. These will contain the group members' best guesses about what activities they would most like to see if more resources were made available to their programme or their sub-programmes (the 'incremental wish list'), and similarly those activities they would be least reluctant to stop if they had a cut in their allocation of resources (the 'decremental wish list'). Second, these wish lists would be costed and assessed in more detail with respect to the impact each listed option would have on benefits. Third, the programme management group would perform the marginal analysis proper where they would assess the impact of shifts of resources of certain amounts, such as £100,000, as they would then have the necessary cost data to do this and as good information as could be made available on the benefit effects.

This economics approach does require data on costs and benefits and it requires that these data relate to changes on the margins of programmes and sub-programmes. To this extent, it might be claimed that the approach is data-intensive. However, I would respond with two arguments: first, any system of priority setting will be data-intensive; second, efficiency of resource use cannot be pursued in practice without information about marginal costs and marginal benefits. Any approach to priority setting that does not involve some assessment of costs and benefits on the margins should be treated with the utmost suspicion.

In the next section, we will look at QALY league tables before turning to other approaches to priority setting and set these in the light of what I have written about the economics approach. However, before doing so I want to highlight the fact that what has been said in this section deals only with efficiency – strictly, allocative efficiency. I have not covered equity. Equity was discussed in detail in Chapter 8, but here it is worth saying that the best way to handle equity in priority setting is perhaps for it to be added on at the end of the efficiency exercise. If the two – efficiency and equity – are considered together, then there is a risk that waters get muddied and there is a loss of clarity with respect to why particular options seem good or bad. Thus, the best way to proceed might be as follows:

First, the authority responsible for the overall running of the services might make a clear statement about what their operational goal for equity is in terms of health, access or use. Thereafter, they might try (but it is difficult) to give guidance as to the relative weight to be attached to equity and in what dimensions: gender, social class and geographical location are the three fairly obvious ones. These equity guidelines would then be presented to the programme management groups to assist them in their deliberations, the idea being that they concentrate initially on efficiency concerns but then indicate what the equity impact would be of the various possible strategies.

When the choices overall come back to the main health service authority from the programme management groups, the final trade-offs between equity and efficiency would be made. Given the inevitably political nature of these choices, it would seem appropriate that these choices with respect to equity are made at this high level.

9.3 QALY league tables

As part of the push for better priority setting, the idea of QALY league tables was developed. These have sparked much interest among policy-makers. Some might even argue that the use of such tables represents *the* way to go in setting priorities. For more detail of QALY league tables, see Gerard and Mooney[2] and Mason et al.[3]

In presenting them here, however, the emphasis is one of caution. Priority setting is hard and fraught with various difficulties and pitfalls. QALY league tables avoid some pitfalls, but they must be used, if at all, with considerable care.

Some overselling of QALY league tables has occurred. There is a risk in this and a need to ensure that expectations with respect to the 'product' are realistic. It is these thoughts that dominate this section.

The middle ground advocated here involves saying yes to QALY league tables with 'large-print warnings' about the sometimes fragile bases for the construction of such tables and fears of overuse and misuse, whilst arguing that PBMA is still the priority-setting technique of choice. At the same time, the middle ground accepts that what currently happens is rather unsatisfactory, that there is considerable room for improvement, and that improvement in the technique of QALY league tables is highly desirable. But it also states that, at a policy level, the principles underlying QALY league tables need to be understood better and applied more widely than is currently the case.

Finally, the middle ground argues strongly that far more important at this stage in the development of priority-setting techniques, and in particular QALY league tables, than improving the QALYs or improving the tables is improving the thinking in priority setting. If there is one thing I would like to change in the armoury of policy-makers, it is how they think about setting priorities. It is getting across strongly to them the concepts of opportunity cost and the margin. Most policy-makers in my experience do not use these simple concepts. Those who are exposed to them have little difficulty in understanding them and readily recognise their relevance to health care planning and priority setting. Some of those who do understand apply them, while others backslide, very often in the face of entrenched disciplinary thinking that has persisted in health care for many years but that nonetheless has been shown to have failed. This backsliding is unfortunate even if understandable. It should stop, and the best way to do this is to sell the economic approach better and to continue to expose the deficiencies of other approaches.

The arrogance of an economist? Yes – and with no apology! For far too long, health care planning has been run by people who do not understand the key concepts involved in priority setting. I can see no reason for trying to defend their position when I am convinced that it is leading to less – and less valued – health in societies than can be the case with no increase in resources at all. While epidemiology is clearly an important discipline in health care planning – and that needs to be emphasised – the philosophy of much of epidemiology is unhelpful when priorities have to be set. While the science of medicine is necessary for understanding disease and reactions of disease to treatments, there is little in the philosophy of medicine that is helpful to priority setting as a process. Other disciplines from the social sciences are also potentially helpful as aids to implementing good priority setting. The key to good priority setting, however, arises from the same source as the discipline of economics – that when there are insufficient resources to do all that we would like to do, then we have to choose how best to use these resources. That is how economics arose as a discipline, and it is from that fact that economics continues to take its lifeblood. Similarly, priority setting in health care exists because resources for health care are scarce and choices have to be made.

A QALY league table is a device or procedure aimed at allowing priority setting of possible changes in health care programmes when these are competing for limited resources, and choices have to be made about where to make changes. The league table ranks different procedures according to the cost per QALY of implementing these procedures. The resource-allocation decision rule underlying the use of these tables is that changes in programmes should be implemented on the rank order basis of ascending cost per QALY.

Strictly, QALY league tables are marginal health service cost per QALY gained league tables (given various assumptions about existing resource allocation and about the objectives that health services are trying to meet in their priority setting). This clarification is important.

First, the fact that QALY league tables are about marginal costs per extra QALY is important. The question arises, margin with respect to what? In other words, from where are we starting? The answer to this is that we are starting from where we are. QALY league tables are based on answers to the question, given the current allocation of resources in a particular area, what are the costs involved in purchasing additional QALYs through the implementation of more of the various procedures that are currently available or through implementing some new procedures altogether? If, say, there is an extra £100,000 to spend on health care, then what is the maximum number of extra QALYs that that can buy? In which procedures is it best to invest more?

It can be anticipated that the cost of buying extra QALYs in a programme will be a function of a number of factors. Almost certainly one of these will be how much of that programme is already being performed. As more and more is invested in a programme, it is likely that the cost per QALY on the margin will rise. This is because it is logical and rational (and efficient) to treat those patients first where the return in terms of QALYs per pound spent is highest and gradually work down to patients where the cost per QALY is getting higher and higher.

It follows that the contents of a QALY league table are a function of what is currently going on within the geographical area for which the priority setting is being done. If, say, a particular health authority has already implemented a sizeable programme of heart transplants, then *ceteris paribus* the marginal cost per QALY of more heart transplants is likely to be higher than in an area that is lagging behind in its heart transplant programme. This is because the first authority will already have given transplants to those patients who are 'good buys' for such a procedure.

A related factor worth noting here is that as, for example, more and more hysterectomies are done, so the cost per QALY within that authority will most likely rise. Thus, if a QALY league table at one point in time within an authority suggests that the lowest cost per QALY lies in the hysterectomy programme, after the authority has invested, say, £100,000 in more hysterectomies, it will be necessary to recalculate the marginal cost per QALY for the hysterectomy programme. If the cost per QALY has changed, then the position of hysterectomies in the QALY league table may also have changed, with the result that, if another £100,000 becomes available, it may not be hysterectomies that are now the 'best buy' for additional QALYs.

Second, the reason why recognition that QALY league tables are about marginal costs per QALY is important is that priority setting here is not about the choice between programmes *per se*. It is about choices between changes in the scale of different programmes.

Beyond the issue of the margin, another important aspect of QALY league tables is that they are about QALYs. Now while that is a rather obvious statement, there is the question of the extent to which QALYs are an accurate and acceptable measure of what is to be measured here. The question becomes: are QALYs an adequate measure of health; or, more accurately, given the marginal nature of such matters, are QALYs gained an adequate measure of health gains? In the context of QALY league tables, it is likely to be the case that for policy-making the QALY is as good a measure of health as is available, and for most purposes in priority setting it is an adequate measure.

What is worth stressing is that QALY league tables are seen as particularly useful in making comparisons across programmes, essentially because the QALY is not programme-specific. It is this broad nature of QALYs that allows the QALY league table to be used in priority setting across surgical, psychiatric, dermatological and many other programmes. If this generality is cast in doubt, then much of the value of the QALY league table would disappear; indeed, it would simply be unworkable. (For a discussion of generic versus condition specific health status measures, see Dowie.[4])

QALY league tables also assume that all that is relevant in the pursuit of priority setting in health care is that health is to be maximised. In so far as other considerations come into play in deciding how best to allocate resources to health and within health care, then QALY league tables will inevitably be deficient. Thus, as discussed in greater length in Chapter 4, if there are other forms of benefit that are relevant in allocating resources – such as information, the protection of autonomy, or whatever – then the use of QALY league tables will lead to some distortions of the 'true' priorities.

Further, QALY league tables are about efficiency – essentially allocative efficiency, i.e. maximising the additional benefit from the additional resources available. They say nothing about equity, except in so far as equity is assumed away by arguing that a QALY is a QALY is a QALY, no matter who receives it, and assuming that equity is to be seen in terms of health and not in terms of access or of use.

The objectives of health care as assumed by QALY league tables are also somewhat problematical on the cost or resource side. On the benefit side, the only benefit allowed is health. This means that, in terms of allocative efficiency, the only form that cost can take legitimately is in terms of opportunity costs, where the benefit foregone is in terms of health. The QALY league table allows the question to be posed: is it better to spend here or there when only health benefits are being assumed?

This seems a reasonable assumption if we accept that health care is only about health for those resources that are within the health care budget. But there are other resources that we would normally want to embrace in any economic evaluation of health care. These would include, for example, the resources of patients and their relatives, those of other social services, such as housing and education services, and so on. But these provide potentially not just health benefits but also other forms of benefit: for the patient, the family and friends, the time input to care might have been used in a very wide range of other activities, from watching TV to climbing mountains; the education services could have been producing more or different forms of education; and so on. The point is simply that these resources from outside the formal health care budget are not restricted in their use and hence in their opportunity costs to health-inducing activities. It is then difficult, indeed impossible, within the constraints imposed by a cost–utility framework to consider non-health service resource use within a QALY league table. It is simply not possible to say that patient time is best spent on this or that treatment, since that judgement can be made only across a much wider range of activities to which that patient time might have been an input.

That means that QALY league tables have to be restricted on the input or resource side in a similar way to that in which they are restricted on the output side, i.e. to health and, with respect to resources, to health service resources that have no alternative use other than the production of health.

These caveats do not mean that we should abandon QALY league tables in priority setting. They are not perfect, and they do have problems, but then so do all the existing approaches to priority setting. At least with QALY league tables some of the key principles of priority setting are adhered to. What does emerge from this discussion is that we need to understand fully what QALY league tables can and cannot do, and that when they are constructed and used they should be treated with caution. Interpretation is crucial. It is the case, however, that PBMA remains the preferred approach.

It can be argued, however, that transfer of effectiveness data, cost data and hence the results of cost–utility studies from one geographical location to another is not appropriate and that it is the results of *local* cost–utility analysis (CUA) studies that should be used in the construction of any QALY league table. In other words, ideally each country, region or area should construct its own QALY league table to reflect the conditions that country, region or area faces locally. Certainly, there is a sense in which that would be ideal, especially if one accepts that the valuation of QALYs may well vary legitimately from one area to another. There is no reason to believe, for example, that the relative weights attached to length of life and all sorts of different forms of quality of life will be constant across different areas of a country, never mind across different countries.

Perhaps this issue is best understood if it is put the other way round. If we were to accept that QALY league tables – the same QALY league table – could be used in Humberside, Hobart, Hamilton and Harare, then this would mean that all these places would have the same priorities for health care, irrespective of how they were currently delivering services and independently of what they were already doing in allocating resources and of what the diseases were and their prevalence in these locations, and how illness and disease were valued in these areas. That seems a most unlikely scenario.

There may be situations where such transfers are both possible and legitimate. This is more likely, for example, in the case of certain forms of drug therapy, where the resource inputs may be very similar from location to location, and where the marginal and average costs may also be similar. But clearly this would apply only to those diseases that existed in the two locations. And, of course, there is the issue of considering how the drug therapies rank vis-à-vis other forms of intervention.

The message here would seem to be not to trust the transfer of results from one location to another until the conditions under which the original study was done are understood and compared with the local situation. Only if these conditions are seen to be reasonably similar should the results from elsewhere be used locally.

Should QALY league tables be constructed? Should they be used? And if so, how and in what circumstances?

The most famous example of the use of QALY league tables arose in Oregon. The aim was to produce a QALY league table for services provided under the state of Oregon's Medicaid programme. The story of Oregon is well documented elsewhere (see, for example, Dixon and Walsh[5]). It remains the case that to have tried this experiment in the USA was a major innovation. Much of the criticism of the Oregon experiment, however, is specific to Oregon rather than to QALY league tables as such. I would therefore not want to use the Oregon experiment to add further criticism to QALY league tables as a device for setting priorities.

The key message with respect to the use of QALY league tables in health care policy-making is that there are advantages in using the tables but that these advantages will be lost if they are not used with care. To date, the extent to which there have been warnings on the packaging about the problems of misuse and overuse has been too little. As a result, there is a danger of policy-makers getting things wrong when using QALY league tables and for the future perhaps becoming disenchanted with the whole idea of priority setting.

PBMA, despite its appearance of being less scientific, remains for the present the preferred approach. QALY league tables handled carefully are useful in priority setting. What is needed to get them used more and better is much more research using CUA and careful use of the thinking underlying QALY league tables.

So this is not a counsel of despair but rather a plea – yet again – for keeping to good principles and using initiative and ingenuity in manipulating data to allow the principles to be applied. That sort of thinking – good principles and pragmatism with data – seems to be emerging as one of the key features of this book.

9.4 Priority setting: some other approaches

A number of other approaches are used in priority setting in health care. These vary from country to country. However, most seem to come under the rather broad heading of 'needs assessment', or variants on this. Here I want to look briefly at needs assessment, target setting as a popular variant of needs assessment, and burden of disease studies. These approaches are reviewed here not with the intent of being comprehensive, but to outline what the main approaches seem to be.

Needs assessment

The most common approach to priority setting would appear to be what is normally referred to as 'needs assessment'. This comes in various guises but in essence involves an attempt to assess the total needs for health care for a population as a whole, or for a particular disease group, or a particular client or age group. This leads into priority-setting exercises, which are initially concerned with assessing the needs for child health services, or for cancer patients, or for elderly people, and perhaps in aggregation for the people as a whole living in a particular location.

The principle lying behind this approach seems to be that the total needs for health care can be established and that somehow this will provide a basis for setting priorities. What is not clear, however (at least to this author), is what one does with the information on needs assessment. If one can establish the total needs for child health care, how do we move forward from that to establish priorities? If the needs for children aged zero to one are greater than for those aged one to two, what does this mean for the allocation of resources between these two groups? If the needs are twice as great, does this mean that resources should be allocated pro rata with the size of the relative needs? Are all needs in this sense weighted equally? In fact, before we can address these sorts of questions, we need to establish what is meant by 'need' in this context.

Need in this context is related directly to illness or sickness. As indicated in Chapter 6, the approach to needs assessment is usually that the more sickness there is in a population, the greater is the need (presumably for health care). Such a view of need would suggest that needs assessment would involve establishing a sickness profile, covering *inter alia* the incidence and prevalence of diseases in the relevant population. It would also be independent, at any moment, of the technological ability to deal with sickness.

If there is a desire to establish the total need for, say, cancer services, then the needs for care for different cancers presumably have to be established and in some way aggregated. But how is this aggregation to be done? One possibility is to establish some sort of indicator, which would reflect the amount of health gain in the community if diseases were eradicated. This might be in terms of something rather crude, like years of life lost prematurely from a disease. Or it might involve an estimate of the burden of disease in terms of, say, total QALYs lost from breast cancer or total QALYs lost from breast cancer among women aged 40 to 50. (Discussion specifically of burden of disease follows later in this chapter.) It might adopt some sort of cost of illness calculation, where the burden of the disease in terms of sickness might be added to the cost of treatment and the costs of lost output in the economy as a result of the disease's existence. But while the literature is not always clear on this point, some measure of need is required and it is presumed here that that measure has to be related in some way to the burden of disease.

There seem to be various possibilities for what to do with this information. One is to argue that resources should be allocated pro rata with needs. The logic here would be that, since this form of needs reflects capacity to benefit, then allocating resources in this way would maximise the amount of need met. But resource use has to reflect the costs of treatment. What about the costs of meeting the needs? It would only be if the cost per unit of need met (perhaps health gain) were constant across all diseases and conditions, and that for all these diseases and conditions average and marginal cost were equal, that this estimate of needs assessed would be valid. That is most unlikely to hold good. Put another way, it would mean that all diseases would be treated in an equally operationally efficient way, i.e. that all diseases were equally cost-effective in their treatment. Further, it would require that technological developments in medicine and in the delivery of health care were such that they did not affect the cost-effectiveness of such treatments at all. It would additionally mean that there were no economies (or diseconomies) of scale for any disease or condition.

A second possibility would be to argue more basically that the needs assessments should be used simply as an ordinal ranking, i.e. that the disease with the greatest needs should get more resources than that with the next greatest need, and so on. In some ways, this is more appealing. However, if the cost-effectiveness of interventions varies, again there is no reason to think that the greatest need should be given priority. Further, if we adopted this ordinal ranking, how would it be used? At what point would we say, that is enough spending on the top need, now let us move to the next? In other words, the lack of cardinality leaves us unable to use the margin in resource-allocation decision-making.

A third possibility is to use the needs assessment information in some form of weighting process, which might reflect priorities. Thus, if it were felt that those diseases or conditions that created the most need in society should be given priority over and above any considerations of some simple cost-effectiveness criterion of allocating resources in such a way as to maximise health gains, then the ranking of needs assessment could be used to arrive at weights. Thus, if, say, cardiovascular disease were the disease for which there was the greatest need, then the health gains from any interventions that had an impact on reducing the needs there might be weighted more highly than those for interventions on other diseases that came further down the needs league table. This was discussed in Chapter 8.

This size of the problem imperative is perhaps understandable in that policy-makers might be attracted by the approach at a superficial level. I cannot see, however, how the approach survives any detailed scrutiny.

On this issue of cost and priority setting, it may be worth repeating why costs are needed in setting priorities. This is because of the concept of opportunity cost. Priority setting is about working out where best to allocate scarce resources, and forming that judgement needs an assessment not only of the benefit of one intervention over another but also an assessment of the costs – the benefits foregone – elsewhere.

If we do not allow for costs in priority setting, this would mean that, if some new technology allowed heart transplants to be carried out at one-tenth of their current cost, then such a change would have no effect on priorities in health care. Again, if the costs of hip replacements rose sixfold, would this not have an effect – *should* this not have an effect – on the level of supply of hip replacements?

Needs assessment leaves this author wondering what there is to gain from any assessment of needs as a totality. It is possible (as discussed in greater length in Chapter 8) that a case can be made for assessing total need in the context of equity. There is no case for total needs assessment exercises for promoting allocative efficiency.

Needs assessment is based on faulty logic – the faulty logic of the imperative of the size of the problem. That faulty logic needs to be exposed – and exposed again.

Explicit choices – even if they are tragic ones – need to be made in health care if priority setting is to help us to arrive at efficient solutions in resource allocation. The dividends from such explicit choices are great and in my view more than enough to justify the extra investment in training and organisational changes that might be required to get decisions faced and to overcome the lack of moral fibre that may hinder better decision-making in health care and that lends support to the needs assessors.

Target setting

There is in itself little wrong with the idea of setting targets in priority setting. Indeed, targets can provide incentives for action and the issue of incentives more generally is one that is somewhat neglected in priority setting. However, very much depends on how the targets are set, and it is here that reservations have to be expressed. The experience to date is not encouraging.

The most famous, or notorious, targets in health and health care were those set by the WHO in their pursuit of the goal of Health For All in the Year 2000. These were, in essence, largely challenges rather than anything more substantial. They were a mixture of concerns for better health, greater equity especially across countries, a desire to involve all sectors of the economy in the provision and promotion of health and not just the formal health care sector, and a large dose of exhortation. They largely failed, although as a source of propaganda for health they may have been effective.

The targets in themselves were fairly harmless. However, the long-term impact might well have been deleterious on three fronts. First, for those countries well below the targets when they were set – Hungary as compared with Sweden, say – there might well have been a concern that there was a lack of understanding in WHO about the differences in all sorts of cultural and economic phenomena that these two countries faced. This could well have had the effect of depressing morale among Hungarian policy-makers – the exact opposite of what the target setters intended. Second, others have followed in the steps of WHO and gone for target setting as a vehicle for health policy. However, at a national level, the sorts of target setting that might have been appropriate for WHO are less likely to be so for a national government, which has at least some executive power to influence what actually happens on the ground.

Third, and in a sense related to the last point, the WHO targets were, in essence, part of their propaganda and sloganising for health. WHO does not have to take responsibility for their implementation. Among national governments, adopting the sloganising approach may well prove counterproductive. There is a responsibility at that level to go beyond slogans and consider operational planning of health care. As a result of the WHO target setting bandwagon, increasingly it seems governments are stepping back from health care policy-making. They set targets and then leave those at the lower echelons of policy-making to determine how the targets are to be reached.

This is heady but very dangerous stuff, because it means that objectives are set without due consideration of means. Goals may be too expensive to achieve. Resource considerations are included too infrequently in the process of target setting. It is words without due consideration of the actions necessary to make the words fulfilling.

Targets are, or ought to be, about allocative efficiency and equity. But at the level of allocative efficiency, objectives and thereby allocative efficiency have to be pursued, taking due account of costs and benefits on the margin. If this is not done, it is difficult to see how allocative efficiency can be advanced. If this process is not adopted in target setting, then there is a very real danger that the targets not only fail to further efficiency but may actually promote inefficiency. In other words, it is not just that they are not 'perfect': they will not be even an approximation to perfection. They are not an approximation in principle, so it is difficult to see how – but for chance – they can result in an approximation in practice in what they can actually achieve.

It is perhaps worth re-emphasising that I do not mean to criticise target setting per se. If targets were set on the basis of weighing up costs and benefits on the margins – as they could be – then I can see considerable merit in them. Certainly, one would want to allow for variations at the local level, and advice and guidance would be needed at the local level about how to use the targets sensibly and flexibly. That is the key merit to target setting, i.e. this visibility in where we want to go, with the visibility allowing goals to be shared, striven for, and so on. But the targets that are used most frequently in health care do not embrace the marginal cost versus marginal benefit principle, so they fail to promote allocative efficiency. It is possible to get the advantages of target setting tied to the advantages of the pursuit of allocative efficiency. Indeed, that is the challenge.

Cost of illness and burden of disease

There is a substantial literature on cost of illness studies where at least a part – and normally a major part – of the defence for doing these studies is that they can be used as a basis for setting priorities. Cost of illness normally covers the costs of treating the illness together with the costs (e.g. from absence from work) arising as a result of the illness. The logic appears to be that, if the costs of a particular illness are high compared with another illness, then the higher-cost illness should get higher priority. To this extent, this is an extension of the needs assessment type of approach. They also cover burden of disease (BOD) studies, which have been popularised and indeed pushed by WHO and the World Bank,[6] and that is at best unfortunate. If I am right in arguing that they are of low or zero value for priority setting, then the fact that WHO has encouraged an army of analysts in developing countries and some developed countries to estimate national burdens of disease has to be worrying. Analytical skills in developing countries are very scarce, and if they are employed in low-value activities the opportunity costs may be very high. Further, it is possible that the results of BOD exercises may actually be used to set priorities in resource allocation, and that is yet more worrying.

What can explain their popularity? This is difficult to answer. There is a superficial attraction, somewhat similar to that in the needs assessment approach, in allocating resources to big problems, but that is so superficial that it is difficult to see that it is the real explanation. Partly, too, it may be that big numbers look impressive, and it may be for this reason that the pharmaceutical industry seems so keen to fund cost of illness studies. I suppose that, if they can show that a disease for which they have a product that will reduce or ameliorate the disease costs a large sum, then this may be a useful advertising weapon. I cannot think that policy-makers would succumb to such an argument, yet it seems that many BOD and cost of illness studies are funded by the pharmaceutical industry, so perhaps there is something in that argument.

It is certainly my view that the use of cost of illness and BOD studies as a basis for priority setting in health care will not lead to an efficient allocation of resources; nor is this a way of getting to something approximating to efficiency. As Davey and Leeder remark in a neat, dismissive and accurate phrase: 'To know the cost of illness is to know nothing of real importance in deciding what we should do about the illness.'[7]

9.5 Conclusion

My prime intention in this chapter was to indicate a simple way in which economic analysis can address the task of priority setting. Also presented was a critique of the potentially useful QALY league tables. I have also indicated that other non-economic approaches are used, but that these remain deficient in certain ways.

How should we judge between different priority setting approaches? There are three questions to ask.

- Does the approach incorporate some assessment of the cost of interventions?
- Does the approach incorporate some assessment of the benefits of interventions?
- Is the approach operating on the margin?

If the answer to even one of these questions is no, then the approach is suspect if efficiency is the goal of priority setting.

I hope to have presented some useful insights into priority setting. I hope, too, that these will be useful both in persuading the reader that the economics approach does have something very positive to offer the priority setters and perhaps also in convincing the reader that other methods fall short in various ways.

I remain somewhat surprised and sometimes a little depressed at how difficult it seems to be to get those concerned with priority setting in health care to accept the economics approach and at the same time to acknowledge the deficiencies of, for example, needs assessment. Perhaps readers of this chapter will see the light.

Questions

1. What is PBMA?
2. Do we need the PB or can we settle for the MA?
3. What would be a more precise name for a QALY league table?
4. What are the pros and cons of needs assessment as a method for priority setting?
5. Is target setting useful in priority setting?
6. Is burden of disease useful? In what context?
7. How best can we judge priority-setting approaches?

Notes

1. C. Mitton and C. Donaldson, 'Twenty five years of programme budgeting and marginal analysis in the health sector', *Journal of Health Services Research and Policy*, 6 (2001), pp 239–248.
2. K. Gerard and G. Mooney, 'QALY league tables: handle with care', *Health Economics*, 2 (1993), pp 59–64.
3. J. Mason, M. Drummond and G. Torrance, 'Some guidelines on the use of cost effectiveness league tables', *British Medical Journal*, 306 (1993), pp 570–572.
4. J. Dowie, 'Decision validity should determine whether a generic or condition specific HRQOL measure is used in health care decisions', *Health Economics*, 11 (2002), pp 1–8.
5. J. Dixon and H.G. Walsh, 'Priority setting: lessons from Oregon', *Lancet*, 337 (1991), pp 891–894.
6. C. Murray, A. Lopez and D. Jamison, 'The global burden of disease in 1990; summary results, sensitivity analysis and future directions', *Bulletin of the World Health Organisation*, 72 (1994), pp 495–509. C. Murray and A. Lopez, 'Progress and directions in refining the Global Burden of Disease approach', *Health Economics*, 9 (2000), pp 69–82.
7. P. Davey and S. Leeder, 'The cost of cost-of-illness studies', *Medical Journal of Australia*, 158 (1993), pp 583–584.

ten

Health care financing and organisation

Health care is about doing better – which means we have to decide the good of health care.

Shane Houston

10.1 Introduction

One of the interesting phenomena in health care in the early twenty-first century is how different the financing and organisation arrangements are in different countries. To describe these and highlight their strengths and weaknesses is not the intention of this chapter. Rather, what I want to do here is to examine why systems differ. This is a mammoth task. Consequently, in order to constrain it and make the process manageable within the space of one chapter, I have chosen to address the question of why a public health service.

Fortunately, while this might appear to have an ideological flavour to it, in practice what emerges are messages for all forms of financing and organisation of health care. The messages are principally about equity in the first place, but they are inevitably, given the links that have been established in earlier chapters, also about ethics and efficiency. What health care services attempt to be efficient about is a function of the ethical and indeed cultural basis of the society. Change the culture, and the ethical base may change, and the goal of efficiency will alter. The key to different health care systems would seem to lie in equity. The question of why a public system is best answered in terms of equity.

In their classic examination of alternative systems of health care provision, three leading British experts – Culyer, Maynard and Williams [1] – suggested that there are essentially two prototypes of systems. There is system X, which:

has as its guiding principle consumer sovereignty in a decentralized market, in which access to health care is selective according to willingness and the ability to pay. It seeks to achieve this sovereignty by private insurance; it allows insured services to be available partially free at time of consumption; it allows private ownership of the means of production and has minimal state control over budgets and resource distribution; and it allows the reward of suppliers to be determined by the market.

Their other prototype, system Y:

has as its guiding principle the improvement of health for the population at large; it allows selective access according to the effectiveness of health care in improving health ('need'). It seeks to improve the health of the population at large through a tax-financed system free at the point of service. It allows public ownership of the means of production subject to central control of budgets; it allows some physical direction of resources; and it allows the use of counter-vailing monopsony power to influence the rewards of suppliers.

They further suggest that it is possible:

to distinguish sharply between two rival ethical bases, on each of which a system of health care can be constructed and justified. The first considers access to health care to be essentially similar to access to all the other good things in society (food, shelter, leisure pursuits); that is, it is part of society's reward system. The second regards access to health care as a citizen's right, like access to the ballot box or the courts of justice, which should not depend in any way on an individual's income and wealth.

I do not want to be critical of this analysis nor of its objectives. Indeed, I think that this particular treatment of the market versus the state debate is much more useful than many of its successors, particularly in respect of treating different systems in their own light. Rather, what I want to pose is an additional question that remains unanswered in the analysis by Culyer and colleagues: why do viewpoints (or ethical bases) vary?

To facilitate understanding of this issue, this chapter concentrates attention on public systems, essentially Y-type systems.

10.2 Key features of public systems

Different writers, politicians, health care commentators and others have put forward their views on what the objectives of public health care systems are, how these differ from others, and why. For example, public systems are more likely to be in the game of promoting universal coverage. There are a number of advantages of such coverage, as Rice indicates:[2]

- Improve the health and productivity of the population by making health services financially accessible to all.
- Obviate the need to provide for a large array of safety-net facilities for uninsured sick people who cannot afford care.
- Cheaper administrative costs because processes such as verifying eligibility for the program will not be necessary.
- Provide government with more clout in keeping provider payments in check.
- Reduce problems of adverse selection into health insurance plans.
- Enhance fairness in society.

Further, it is important to recognise in this context two other things. First, there is no reason to believe that different countries will subscribe to the same health care goals. Second, funding health services differently inevitably means a different value base on which to build health care.

With respect to the first point, this seems very obvious. Yet the WHO World Health Report suggests that all health care systems across the world will have and should have the same goals.[3] Not just that; the goals such as equity will be defined in the same way and will be given the same relative weight in all countries.[4] WHO argues that to assess a health system 'one must measure five things: the overall level of health; the distribution of health in the population; the overall level of responsiveness; the distribution of responsiveness; and the distribution of financial burden'. For each, different types of data are needed for each country to calculate measures of attainment. The implication is that the objectives of all health systems can be measured in terms of increases in and the distribution of disability-adjusted life expectancy (DALE), improved levels of and the distribution of responsiveness, and the fair distribution of the financing burden. It is claimed that, since a system can do well on some dimensions and poorly on others, comparison across countries or through time requires that the five measures be aggregated together. A weight reflecting relative importance is assigned to each. This provides an overall attainment score for each health system. This will enable some ranking of countries in terms of how well they perform. A second measure of performance is proposed that relates overall attainment to the availability of resources.

Why, however, would one expect or want to apply a common set of values across different countries? Where is the recognition that preferences may vary across different countries? As any basic summary measure of health is extended to include other factors, no matter how desirable this might be in principle, the prospects of its applying within a common set of values across different cultures would seem to diminish. For example, equity can be viewed in different ways and in turn the extent to which different cultures value equity also varies. There is the yet more fundamental question of whether all health services subscribe to the same set of goals.

As Rice argues:[5]

> Different countries may not want the same things from their health care systems. Some may want to emphasize access, others cost control, others efficiency over equity, and still others the opposite. Moreover, historical and cultural factors are critical determinants of how different countries' health services systems have developed, making it risky to suggest that any one country's system be replicated by others.

He goes on: 'Creating an agreed-upon set of weights among the different outcomes would probably be impossible. How does one weigh, for example, the short waits (a characteristic of the U.S. system) against the equity of health system financing (a characteristic of the U.K. system)?'

These comments are intended to encourage readers at least to reflect critically on the concepts of universalism in preferences for health and on the relevant constructs of health. What is at stake is in essence three things. First, what are the objectives of each health care system? There is no reason to believe that once we move beyond a rather vague goal of the promotion of the health of the population that all countries will adopt the same objectives. Second, what (and whose) values are to be used to determine the relative weights to be attached to the different components of the objectives of health care systems? Third, who is to determine whose preferences are to be used? There is no reason to believe that there will be universal answers to these three questions.

It could be considered that one advantage of a public system is that it might place less responsibility (or, in a sense, cost) on the individual in making choices. Choice would seem to be greater in the private sector than in the public sector. Indeed, this greater freedom of choice is often put forward as a plus for the private sector.

It is far from clear, however, that at the level of the individual, as opposed to the community at large, the individual is less or more able to avoid difficult decisions or to abrogate personal responsibility for decision-making under a public as opposed to a private system. Given the agency relationship, such avoidance is not only possible but present under all systems of health care; it appears to be a function of uncertainty regarding illness episodes and treatment availability and effectiveness, and the expected loss if things do go wrong. It is not immediately apparent that any one system is better at reducing uncertainty than any other, except perhaps that under at least some public systems there is greater certainty of access to health care. The probability of things going wrong may be a function of the system in so far as the effectiveness of care is a function of the system. But the evidence on this is very weak indeed.

Much depends here on what sorts of choices are at stake and whether the choices involved are truly individual. This issue is picked up again in the final chapter of this book.

Rather than conjecture more generally about the objectives of public systems, we can look at the evidence of history. On the basis of what public systems do, do they reveal their preferences? Can we, through their behaviour, spot what it is that they have been trying to achieve?

Some potentially key concerns of health care systems are:

- technological innovation
- equity geographically, by social class
- effectiveness
- efficiency
- professional status
- patients' rights/preferences
- clinicians' rights
- the community's preferences
- medical ethics/clinical freedom.

This list is incomplete. On some counts, it is impossible at present to make truly informed judgements about strengths and weaknesses across different systems, often because of measurement problems (e.g. effectiveness and consequently efficiency). With others, system and affluence tend to get clogged up together as, for example, in the case of technological innovation. Others again seem remarkable in their similarity. As Veatch suggests, medical ethical codes may vary (but it seems not markedly) simply because of different methods of organising and financing health care.[6]

We are left with equity variables, professional status and individual patients' versus the community's rights/preferences – all related to each other since some emphasis on one will tend to mean less weight elsewhere in terms of the values that drive the system. The less sovereign the individual consumer, the higher is professional status. These will be influenced in turn by the community's values, although potentially in different directions. This phenomenon was apparent in the reforms in the 1990s in the UK and New Zealand, where attempts to strengthen consumer choice met with some opposition from the medical profession. The more potent the community feeling, the more concern, *ceteris paribus*, will there be with equity. Given the central importance of the potency of the community feeling, equity and the relationship between these, the rest of this chapter will be devoted to these issues.

Equity, as highlighted in Chapter 8, can be and has been defined in many ways in health care. All of the definitions identified have equality in common; most are dependent on defining need in some way or other; all have been the subject of some confusion.

It is difficult to determine which, if any, of them is in any sense the 'right' definition. Clearly, such a judgement is value-laden, unless, of course, it is already laid down in law or custom that some lexicographic priority is to be given to equity over all other possible goals or objectives.

An important value judgement here relates to the relative weight to be attached to equity vis-à-vis efficiency. For example, equality of access for equal need, if pursued in full, will result almost inevitably in inefficiency in the sense of less health being provided than could be from the resources available; for example, providing sophisticated inpatient care in all areas of a country will promote more equal access but potentially less health for a given budget.

These issues were dealt with in detail in chapter 8. Here, I want to consider more fundamentally the question raised earlier in this chapter of why the viewpoints on which health care systems are based differ, with the focus here specifically on the community's preferences and the weight attached to equity.

10.3 Fair shares for all?

Normally, the expression 'fair shares for all' is thought of in terms of the distribution of some set of goods or services that is declared just in terms of society at large or some sub-group. It is thus about giving out good things fairly.

In an interesting (but for some readers a potentially difficult) and path-breaking way of thinking about social policy, Margolis[7] (and later Sen[8] and Mooney[9]) turned around this standard way of viewing fair shares for all. Margolis considers fair-sharing as not what one gets but what one does; that is, he sees it as doing one's fair share rather than getting one's fair share. He seizes on the fact that we are all, to a greater or lesser extent, social and political animals and that we view ourselves not just as individuals with the ability to enjoy the good things of this life. Additionally, we want to do our fair share for the society, the community, the group, the family – at least some set of individuals wider than but including our individual selves.

The motivation for this willingness to do our bit is not based on the output from our actions in helping or assisting the group; it is the action per se that generates the utility that serves as the motivation. It is the knowledge that we are participating that counts.

Altruism? Perhaps, but not in a pure form, since Margolis stresses that, in participating in the group and devoting resources to the group, we as individuals are equal members of the group. Also, the motivation is not strictly or directly to help others. It is not so much feeling useful as feeling good through group participation.

His fair-shares model is developed in the context of social policy generally. Here, I want to describe his approach in some detail and then show how it applies to health care – indeed, how it applies better to health care than other rationales for equity that have been proposed. Thereafter, I want to draw some conclusions based on the explanatory power of Margolis' model.

The basic postulate on which Margolis builds his approach is that individuals obtain utility (satisfaction) in two ways: first in the normal (economic) sense of getting satisfaction from the goods and services that we consume – the form of utility we encountered in Chapter 2 in the explanation of demand; second – and this is the novel aspect – through participation in group-oriented activities. The utility derived from this group-related activity is not directly a function of either the utility of the output the individual receives as an equal member of the group or the utility of the output that the group receives. However, the willingness of individuals to participate is, in part, a function of the degree of efficiency with which the group-oriented activities are organised as perceived by the individual. In other words, individuals are more willing to take part in efficient groups or efficient group activities than inefficient ones. Thus, the utility in this second form is process rather than output utility: it is the doing rather than what is given or received that counts.

The individual splits their resources between activities through which they obtain utility selfishly and those through which they obtain utility as a result of participating in the group. As is usual in utility theory, the individual attempts to maximise utility; which means ensuring that the sum of the selfish utility and group-participation utility is the greatest possible. Thus, if the individual can get even greater utility from using some of their resources to participate more in group-oriented activities than spending them on themselves, then they will do so. Such switches of resources will continue until the individual cannot increase their total utility any more. At this point, they will have the optimum balance between their allocations to the self and to the group.

Unless pure altruism lies behind fair-sharing, then the least selfish individuals in society run the risk of being exploited by the more selfish. The likelihood of this is, of course, dependent on the different degrees of selfishness that individuals have within the group (or society). If all are equally selfish (and hence equally selfless), then there will be no exploitation and a stable situation will obtain. However, this is most unlikely. How, then, can the potential for exploitation be removed or reduced?

Margolis suggests that his participation ratio, which is a function of the ratio of spending to obtain group participation utility and spending to obtain selfish utility, would not be constant for each individual. Rather, it would vary in that the more an individual had already allocated to the group, the less they would want to participate still more in the group.

Although that is in essence what the fair-shares model is about, for those interested it is worth expanding the explanation a little more through the use of two diagrams. On the vertical axis in Figure 10.1 are measured the marginal utility of the individual's allocation to themselves, S', and the marginal utility, as perceived by the individual, of the group's spending, G' (not of the individual's allocation to the group). On the horizontal axis is the individual's resource allocation to selfish activities (i.e. s, which has a maximum value of I, the individual's income).

It should be noted in Figure 10.1 that, as the individual devotes more and more of their resources to selfish ends (i.e. as s moves outwards towards I), there is no impact on G'. However, G' is influenced by the individual's perception of the marginal utility to the group (of which the individual is an equal member) of the aggregate resources for group interest. Thus, G_1' is higher than G_2' because, independently of their contribution to the group, the individual perceives the marginal productivity of the group's resources to be higher in the former case than the latter. (If you have a choice of contributing to one of two organisations, one of which you perceive as being efficient and the other inefficient, *ceteris paribus*, which will you choose?)

In Figure 10.2, the key to the model is contained in the two functions presented there. First, G'/S', the value ratio, is the ratio of marginal G-utility as perceived by the individual and marginal S-utility to the individual. Now, from Figure 10.1 we know that G' is unaffected by the individual's allocation between group and self-interest, but S' is affected: as the individual devotes more and more of their income to self-interest, so the marginal utility of their self-interested activities will fall. (This is based on the simple principle introduced in Chapter 2 of diminishing marginal utility, i.e. the more you have, the less you value an extra unit.) Consequently, as the individual devotes more and more of their income to selfish ends (i.e. as s moves closer to I), so S' will fall and, since G' is constant throughout, G'/S' will rise, as in Figure 10.2. The participation ratio, W, is wholly a function of the act of participating. Utility here is in the act, not the outcome. But the more the individual acts in the group interest – that is, the more of their income they devote to the group

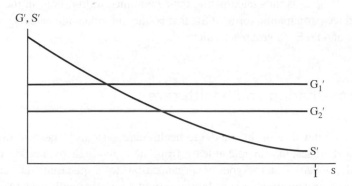

Figure 10.1 Marginal utility (G') of the group's resources allocated to group interest and marginal utility (S') of Smith's resources allocated to selfish interest (s), s + g = I, g = Smith's allocation to the group and I = Smith's income

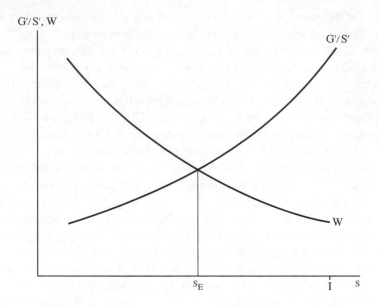

Figure 10.2 Equilibrium of G'/S' and W

– the less is the marginal utility of devoting still more. Consequently, as the individual devotes more and more to selfish ends (and less and less to group ends), so the participation ratio, which is a function of the ratio of the individual's spending on group participation utility and spending on S-utility, will fall.

The individual is thus maximising their combined utility, both in the S-utility form and the participation form, at S_E; that is, the individual allocates S_E to selfish activities and $I - S_E$ to group activities.

10.4 Fair-sharing and health care

What is the relevance of this model to health care systems? These sit on a spectrum that stretches, in principle at least, from the individualistic, market-oriented, part-of-the-reward-system type of organisation to a paternalistic, equitable, needs-based organisation. What Margolis' model does is to allow us to see these different systems in the dimensions of group-participation utility and selfish utility. Thus, to the extent that a society is composed of individuals who find their equilibrium between selfish utility and group participation to be very much at the selfish utility/low participation end, then it will be the market-oriented system of health care that will dominate. If individuals are of the type who are keen to participate and play down selfish utility, then the UK NHS-type system will more likely obtain.

In 1970, Titmuss published his book *The Gift Relationship*, which showed that supplying blood through a process of voluntary donation (as in the UK) was more effective and almost certainly more efficient than the commercial process used in the USA.[10] While the empirical evidence seemed to support him on this front, it was the wider aspects of his book (subtitled *From Human Blood to Social Policy*) that provoked greater controversy and that make it a classic. He wrote: 'Altruism in giving to a stranger does not begin and end with blood donations. It may touch every aspect of life ... it is likely that a decline in the spirit of altruism in one sphere of human activities will be accompanied by similar changes in attitudes, motives and relationships elsewhere.'

It was from this sentiment that Titmuss went on to describe the establishment of the UK NHS in the following terms: 'The most unsordid act of British social policy in the twentieth century has allowed and encouraged sentiments of altruism, reciprocity and social duty to express themselves; to be made explicit and identifiable in measurable patterns of behaviour by all social groups and classes.'

Despite his protestation, it is clear that Titmuss saw the UK NHS as a morally superior form of organisation of health care, not primarily because of what it delivers by way of health but what it does to promote altruism. Whatever one's views are on whether to support Titmuss in these conjectures, in terms of justifying the NHS it would be unfortunate if we had to rely solely on the argument that, whatever its merits in terms of health, it was better at delivering altruism. Where does this leave Margolis? It is likely that Margolis would endorse the idea that the NHS represents a means whereby the community can pass to a single body the responsibility for the community's health. On the notion of the caring externality, there is a parallel with the idea of group utility. However, the issue of participation seems to win in practice in that the evidence supports the view that the NHS's equity goal is couched in terms of access rather than health or, indeed, health care consumption. Access for the group is essentially what Margolis is about: beyond that utilisation and health involve selfish utility resources, a point that appears to be accepted at least implicitly in NHS policy.

Margolis is at pains to point out that he is not concerned with any ethical aspect with which some might imbue his fair-shares model but simply how well it explains how people behave. Margolis is thus set firmly in utilitarianism.

I would therefore conclude on the basis of this discussion that the factor that primarily separates out different health care systems is equity, defined probably in terms of some concept of equality of access. Where participation altruism *à la* Margolis is strong and there is a relatively homogeneous set of preferences in a society, then the health care financing system is likely to be at the more publicly funded end of the spectrum. Where concern for individual utility is of prime interest to the citizens of a country, and freedom of choice fosters heterogeneity of preferences, more market-oriented health care systems will tend to prevail. It is not a complete explanation by any means but, looking at the UK and Denmark on the one hand and the USA on the other, would seem to provide some empirical support for this explanation of why health care financing systems differ.

10.5 Other insights from Margolis

This section discusses briefly two other aspects of Margolis' model which seem to provide useful insights into the nature of health care systems: isn't the caring externality enough? is fair-sharing different?

If individuals care about others in the sense of caring about their access to health care, can we not replace fair-sharing with this caring externality? Certainly, caring about access and fair-sharing are very similar, but caring about access might not get us beyond compulsory health insurance for all. Also, the notion of fair-sharing can be explained more satisfactorily (wanting to do my bit for my fellow person, provided they do their bit for me) than can the caring externality. In the context of our attitudes to self-induced disease (e.g. smoking-induced bronchitis), fair-sharing seems a more appropriate base for the analysis than the caring externality. The latter appears incapable of distinguishing one bronchitic from another; the former can because of the concern permitted about exploitation of the group interest – essentially, here, the fact that as a result of one individual's over-indulgence in selfish interest (i.e. smoking) the costs may fall on the group, and the community's G-interest may thereby be diminished.

Strictly, too, fair-sharing does not involve any externality at all. This is because the utility derived by individuals outside of selfish utility is through participation. Thus, total utility is the sum of all individuals' selfish utilities plus the sum of all individuals' utilities derived from participating in the group. To include the utility derived by the group from the resources allocated to the group (which is what the externality would normally be considered to be) would involve an element of double counting.

Potentially this gets us back into the debate (see Chapter 3) about whether, in what ways and to what extent health care is different from other commodities. The 'whether' question seems to be answered yes, given the extent of the empirical evidence showing that health care markets do seem to be rather different from others. Regarding the question 'in what ways?', the key elements I would suggest are two and related: first, consumers' lack of knowledge of the commodity and, second, the near-monopoly position of the medical profession regarding this very same knowledge. One way of acknowledging the potential for problems in this asymmetric world of knowledge is to have the state as the final arbiter with respect to the profession controlling information in health care (i.e. the medical profession). As individuals, we are ignorant with regard to health care, therefore we are weak. This can be dealt with in one of two ways. First, attempt to strengthen the power of the consumer through increased competition. Clearly something can be done to give consumers better information – but not sufficiently in my view, or at least not sufficiently to allow us to have it at a cost that would make the process worthwhile. Consequently, the second approach seems preferable. Our best defence is in the power of the state; hence nationalisation. The question of 'to what extent?' is a cultural value judgement. The greater is this concern to control the medical profession – the more often the question *'quis custodiet ipsos custodes?'* ('who guards the guardians?') is posed – the less market regulation is accepted as a feasible solution, and the greater the homogeneity of values in a society, the more likely the health service will be nationalised.

These arguments could be extended. Yet there seems enough here to believe that the Margolis model can go a long way to help to explain not only the structure of different health care systems but also why they differ in different societies.

10.6 Which system?

As indicated, systems of health care are or should be culturally based. What is meant by health varies culturally and even within countries (such as, in Australia, between Aboriginal people and non-Aboriginal people). In addition to health, what different societies want from their health care system is also likely to vary. How different cultures want health care delivered will differ. There is no universally best health care system, and searching for it is a waste of time.

Nevertheless, what does become clear is that the push to standardise health care systems, as comes from WHO and the attempts to ape facets of other countries' systems (especially those of the USA and the UK in Diagnosis Related Groups (DRGs) funding of hospitals, Oregon's priority-setting approach, and the internal market), may well be misplaced. This is not to argue for isolationism in thinking about health care planning and systems design. Lessons can be learned from other countries. To argue, however, that Denmark's health care problems and the solutions to these problems are likely to be very Danish is where to start, rather than looking for universal problems and universal solutions. Most countries have some unique health problems, often unique health care issues, and most often unique health care solutions. Learning from others is fine as long as it is not a substitute for thinking through one's own problems and solutions. What is best for the USA is unlikely to be best for Uruguay, the UK or Uganda. The emphasis on equity in the Scandinavian countries may well not suit US values.

Yet having said that, some issues are clear. If countries do want to pursue equity in health care, that is achieved more easily under a publicly funded system than under either a private or mixed system. If individual freedom of choice is weighted highly, then private is to be preferred. If medical power is to be constrained within a more community-based approach, then public is more likely to be the answer. If there is an acceptance that choice is to be exercised by those who can, but the disadvantaged are to be protected by some safety net, then mixed is the answer.

What seems almost unanswerable – and this is frustrating (at least for this author) – is that it is so difficult to judge what the most efficient road is. To some extent, this is understandable once it is accepted that systems are not neutral with respect to what efficiency is about. There are arguments that the incentives of private systems probably enhance the prospects for delivering technical efficiency. Similarly, if done well, in the sense of reflecting public values better, public systems have a greater potential for delivering allocative efficiency. It is not, however, a matter of tossing a coin. What seems increasingly important yet too little researched or even considered is to establish the goals of health care systems. It is this oft-neglected issue that is dealt with in the concluding chapter of this book.

The message from this chapter is simple: if we are to provide better health care systems, we need to agree that a definition of what is 'good' is needed before we get to 'better'. So much planning in health care, economic and other, seems to be based on data and data manipulation rather than good thinking. I have said before that, while medicine is about doing good, economics is about doing better. Here, the issue is what good health care seeks to achieve and how economics can then help to do this better.

A colleague in Perth, Shane Houston, asked to rewrite a draft of a health department statement on strategic planning, called it 'doing better'. That is what health care systems seek to do. That is the message from this chapter.

Questions

1. What are the supposed advantages of public health care systems?
2. And of private systems?
3. And of mixed systems?
4. Do all countries want the same from their health care systems?
5. What is participation utility? How does it relate to equity?
6. What can we learn from other countries' systems?
7. Should we settle for doing good?

Notes

1. A.J. Culyer, A. Maynard and A. Williams, 'Alternative systems of health care provision: an essay on motes and beams', in *A New Approach to the Economics of Health Care*, ed. M. Olson (American Enterprise Institute: Washington and London, 1981), p 134.
2. T. Rice, *The Economics of Health Care Reconsidered* (Health Administration Press: Chicago, 2002).
3. World Health Organization, *The World Health Report 2000* (WHO Publications: Geneva, 2000).
4. G. Mooney and V. Wiseman, 'World Health Report 2000: challenging a world view', *Journal of Health Services Research and Policy*, 5 (2000), pp 198–199.
5. T. Rice op. cit.
6. R.M. Veatch, *A Theory of Medical Ethics* (Basic Books: New York, 1980).
7. H. Margolis, *Selfishness, Altruism and Rationality* (Cambridge University Press: London, 1982).
8. A. Sen, *Inequality Re-Examined* (Clarendon Press: Oxford, 1992).
9. G. Mooney, 'Communitarianism and health economics', in *The Social Economics of Health Care*, ed. John Davis (Routledge, London, 2001).
10. R.M. Titmuss, *The Gift Relationship* (Allen and Unwin: London 1970).

eleven

Some future roads to travel?

Quis custodiet ipsos custodes?

11.1 Introduction

Where does this leave us? Basically in something of a turmoil is the most accurate answer. In many ways, economics is the dismal science in that its analysis of health care is far from joyous.[1] But the silver lining is that, if the will is there, the situation can be improved through the use of economics.

Beyond the ideas put forward in the previous chapter, I have endeavoured to avoid the polemics of the collectivist versus the market debate. For the majority of practitioners, that in any case is not the issue. All systems have their inefficiencies in practice; all systems are capable of being made more efficient and almost certainly, where desired, more equitable.

What is increasingly important is that, following the flurry of systems activity in the latter part of the twentieth century, there is a growing recognition that there is no universal grand design. In the wake of 'following in father's footsteps' – father, here, being some other country and very often the USA or the UK – on so many aspects of other countries' health care systems approaches, there is a greater readiness to look at what individual countries want from their health care systems. At the same time, WHO does the world a disservice and most certainly the developing world by pushing for a world ranking of health care systems based on common features that WHO defines and then endorses.[2]

It is this issue – what health care systems are about and the values they are based upon – that I want to work towards in this final chapter. It is unlikely that readers will need to be persuaded of the reasons why, as a health economist, I would seek to discuss this and yet more importantly have it discussed. If efficiency and equity, which are revealed as the two main pillars of health economics and of health care systems, are to be addressed satisfactorily, then the basis on which they are to be built needs to be examined. What are the benefits that are to be maximised from health care systems? How most equitably should health care resources be deployed? Who should best answer these questions? How can information on such matters best be elicited?

Additionally, I want to write a little about where health economics is and where I believe it is going or ought to go in the coming years. Such comments seem appropriate at the end of a book that has been, by and large, singing the praises of this sub-discipline of economics. Is such singing merited?

By now, it should be clear to the reader that, if they are interested in the pursuit of a healthy population and a fair distribution of health (or access to health care) within that population, then economic analysis, in principle at least, is on the side of the angels. In practice, and in its frequent misuse, it is not surprising that economics gets a bad press in health care. This is largely the fault of economists. Beyond that, the faults for what is currently happening lie elsewhere.

Too often, as societies, we have got health care policy wrong. Much depends on the expectations of the public; this varies from country to country. Yet little is done in any country to adjust the public's expectations to more reasonable levels. Much also depends on the medical profession; this seems to vary little from country to country. We need to do more to restrain in particular the acute clinicians, especially in their resource-unconstrained endeavours. We can do without the caricature of the clinician, armed with the sword of clinical freedom, and clothed in the armour of self-righteousness, protected (from serious thought processes) by the mythical shield of infinite resources, attempting to save the world from death and disease. We can and should respect their skills in the operating theatre and the intensive care unit, but it is less apparent that we should laud them if they attempt to lead the charge on the way to health for all. Of course, doctors have a right to promote health care and to give hope to their patients. As they do so, however, it is worth noting that they may not do so solely for reasons of altruism.

The medical profession has a tendency to see the battle against death and disease as to be fought almost exclusively within the walls of the major teaching hospitals. Again, the inability of clinicians to see the opportunity cost in a wider context is to some extent understandable. It is, however, not acceptable that society's representatives, be they politicians or public officials, do not see opportunity cost in its social or as a minimum wider health service context. Quite how best to ensure that the distribution of property rights (as economists describe the phenomenon) or power more crudely can be altered to ensure that social goals are implemented is a major issue. It is possible for the economist to back off at this point and argue that their task is done when the evaluation or analysis is written up.

That is not good enough, and some recent work in economics using political economy and institutionalist economics (see, for example, Jan[3]) suggests that getting change in the system can be, and perhaps also should be, part of the task of economists. A way forward specifically on this front is outlined later in this chapter. Equity in health care means much more to society at large than to doctors. Certainly, it comes at a cost. But in the context of health care, is the opportunity cost of greater equity really too high? Has the last 0.5 per cent of gross national product (GNP) devoted to supposedly better health been justified rather than being devoted to more equal access? I don't know the answers to these questions. My point is that we need more often to get round to posing them.

In this concluding chapter, I want to spell out some of the ways that, as an economist, I consider might be pursued to try to ensure more efficient, equitable health care. There is no single solution, but getting widespread agreement to an objective of fair and efficient delivery of health for the community would get us quite a long way down the road towards a solution.

11.2 Education

It is wrong to blame the people in the health care system for their lack of use of economics and understanding of this discipline if they have never been taught even the basics. Daily, the health service journals, health policy statements and health care plans abound with misperceptions about and lack of awareness of things economic. Worse, there is a downright distrust and suspicion of this noble discipline, especially among clinicians.

Clearly, these attitudes have to be changed, and where better to start than with undergraduate medical education? In all health care systems, doctors, especially hospital clinicians, have to be managers, even if many of them do not appreciate the fact. Yet the extent to which they are trained in management skills, such as economics, is minimal.

In teaching economics to medical students, a frequent response is: 'It's not us you want to get at, it's the consultants.' Agreed; but how do we get at the consultants? This is not a rhetorical question. There is a need to educate consultants in some basic economics. Perhaps first, however, there is a need to sell them economics. Once some of the medical profession get themselves to the top of the ladder, when there is no longer any risk in climbing, they can and do act as excellent salespeople for economics – especially to their fellows in the medical trade.

There is little reason why just a little economics could not be taught in all medical schools as a compulsory, examinable subject. Certainly, no senior registrar should be allowed to take up a consultant post without some knowledge, from, say, a one-week course in economics. For someone about to run a business with a turnover of almost certainly well in excess of £0.5 million a year, a minimum of one week's compulsory training in economics would not go amiss.

But education should not stop at the medical profession. Most senior nurses in my experience are already skilled in amateur economics. At least they are aware of the principles and the practice of trying to do the best they can with the resources available. They need more formal training, especially before entering management; but in terms of their awareness, and amenability to learn economics, they are some way ahead of most of their medical colleagues.

Administrators and finance staff often have some knowledge of economics. It is usually less than is adequate for the tasks they face. Health service management – and this seems to be an international problem – is low in status, requisite skills and appropriate training. A training in economics cannot solve all these deficiencies, but there are worse places to start.

Perhaps most important of all, there are people – the public at large, the patients and the politicians. For all these groups, there is a general need for health service education in order to allow reality to win in health care debates. Such health service education needs some basis in economics.

Finally, there is a need to educate economists. In all countries, there is a shortage of trained health economists. We need more of them. The best way to get our fellow economists interested is to offer them the right incentives.

This shortage of health economists is a problem. While health planners and managers increasingly seek economists' advice and more health service personnel apply for courses in health economics, the supply of health economists expands all too slowly. There has been a shift in the past few years, with the UK and Canada showing the way. Australia, on the other hand, remains incredibly backward in health economics, on both the supply side and the demand side. There is a need for more undergraduate exposure to health economics in economics faculties and more widespread opportunities to train in health economics at a postgraduate level.

11.3 Information

In most public systems, there is little information available to key decision-makers on costs and little evaluation is conducted. One can also question whether there is good information available on the effectiveness side in either public or private systems. Evidence-based medicine (EBM) is helping on this front, as discussed later. Certainly, where there is a billing system either to the patient or a third-party payer, information on costing tends to be better; on evaluation and outputs, there are few if any systems that do enough.

Information, cost-consciousness, monitoring of performance and standards, evaluation of care, planning – all are poor in most systems, largely because there are few incentives to do better. There is little point in economists indulging in beating doctors over the head because of their inefficiencies if the doctors do not have the information available on which they themselves can judge their efficiency.

Providing cost information alone, unless it affects the doctor directly, will have little effect on doctor efficiency. This is understandable. To expect otherwise can only be as a result of a false understanding of what constitutes appropriate cost information. It is not particularly informative to tell a young child that they cannot have a lollipop because it costs £1. Tell them that they can have two ice-creams for the price of this lollipop and they'll get the message very quickly. So cost information per se is not the answer; it is awareness of opportunity cost that matters. That has to be the message of exercises to provide cost information. Related to this is the fact that cost information in a no-choice situation is, at best, irrelevant and, at worst, confusing. Even in a choice situation, as indicated in Chapter 2, it is necessary to ensure that we have got the *right* cost information.

To place all the emphasis on cost information would, however, play into the hands of those who think that economics is only about costs and cutting costs. Just as important, for those who understand the concept of opportunity cost, is the output or benefit side. It is here – as discussed in Chapter 4 – that the real challenge of measurement lies. It would help even more if the scientific journals and, before them, the research funders took a much more rigorous line in vetting research and its findings. It is not good enough to know that method A diagnoses better than method B. We want to know how much better and what the implications are for treatment and thereby health status as a result of better diagnosis. Nor is it enough to know that cancer patients treated with chemotherapy have a 50 per cent chance of survival for five years. What we want to know is what effect, impact for change, the treatment has – and not just on life expectation. So much could be done here, but so little is. Even the little that is done seems to be ignored too often.

Output at the clinical level can be measured better, as can effectiveness. And not just at the clinical level. Outputs can often be measured in terms of mortality and morbidity; when it proves impossible to do so, let's use informed corporate guesses (often called 'consensus conferences'). I would rather be operated on on the basis of an informed guess made corporately by the medical profession as a whole or general surgeons as a whole or neurosurgeons as a whole than on the guess, even informed, of one individual surgeon. The situation here is improving as a result of EBM and meta-analyses. The remaining problem here relates more to incentives to get change effected and to extend measurement beyond health (as discussed in Chapter 4).

One particularly important issue with regard to clinical decision-making that has become of increased significance in recent years is that of medical practice variations. There are enormous variations geographically in the rates at which various common procedures are conducted. These variations are the result of various influences. What is very clear is that a large part is due to differences in the way that doctors practise. Doctors simply do not agree as to what is best medical practice. While in economic terms best medical practice ought to be equated with efficient practice (with some allowance for equity), it is not at all clear from the literature what the medical criteria are for defining best medical practice. Given the lack of knowledge (even if not their fault) of doctors of the costs of their activities and the apparent lack of knowledge of the effectiveness of their treatments, or at least disagreement about effectiveness, it is hardly surprising that such variations in medical practice exist. It is surprising that the variations are allowed to continue, however. It is a situation that we would not accept from our plumbers, and one that most doctors would not accept from their secretaries.

Yet knowledge of these variations is not new. It has existed for over 50 years. The problem, however, as Evans has described it, is simple. 'Knowing is not the same as doing.'[4] This is the nub. There is here a serious problem for all health care services, and it is a problem that, although it originates with medical science, is then, in terms of its continuance, the responsibility of policy-makers and politicians. It is they who must try to ensure the effective and efficient use of society's scarce resources in health care. While practice guidelines can help, simply announcing these is not enough. They must be accompanied by incentives to change.

There is also the issue of management information. Giving out cost information to clinicians has been tried in a number of countries. Can we not learn internationally from that? Measuring effectiveness of clinical treatments is an international industry, information about which is unconstrained by national boundaries. Measuring effectiveness of management 'treatments' is similarly an international industry, yet many managers appear not to know what is going on even in the adjoining health authority and show little interest in looking to other countries. However, there are signs of change for the better in this respect.

Finally, a word is appropriate about too much information or using information as a substitute for thought. An enormous amount of routine data is collected in all health care systems. Yet when I go to look for information relevant to some specific problem I am analysing, more often than not I find I have to generate my own data. Am I alone? I don't think so, and consequently a note of caution is relevant. There is a need to monitor collected data routinely to see whether anyone is actually using them for some good purpose. If not, then do the data need to be collected routinely at all? All data collection has a cost; that cost needs to be weighed up against the added value and probability of its use. This happens too infrequently. Information also ought to be seen as an aid to planning, evaluation and management and not as a substitute for these. There has to be a good case for thinking about what is to be done with data before collecting them. This might lead to the collection of different data, or fewer or more data. I would therefore not want my plea for more information to be taken as a blank cheque for health care information systems officers to extend their empires without thought for either the cost or the benefit of their activities. A particularly good (or bad?) example of this phenomenon is the issue of needs assessment, which has become public health's main pillar in so many planning and priority-setting exercises in health care. It is an issue that was discussed in some detail in Chapter 9.

11.4 Evaluation and monitoring

Evaluation and monitoring may simply be other forms of information, but the issues surrounding them seem sufficiently important to warrant a separate section on their own. One problem here is that the words themselves mean all things to all people. 'Evaluation', to me, means four things:

- Is this worth doing in terms of doing any good? Is it effective?
- Is it worth doing it this way rather than that? What is more cost-effective?
- Is it worth doing, given the opportunity cost involved? Are the benefits greater than the costs?
- Is it worth doing more? Are the benefits of more greater than the costs of more?

Monitoring means checking afterwards to see whether what was thought before turned out to be right – and if not, then why not. Consequently, monitoring can lead to not just seeing whether we got it right but also increasing the probability of getting it more right in the future through improving our evaluation methods.

Unfortunately, many clinical evaluations seem to address the wrong question, or at least questions that are focused too narrowly. Perhaps this is understandable. More money needs to be made available for studies in evaluation and monitoring, but unless the money and the research are heavily policed, then more (if it comes from a vested interest like the drug industry) will not automatically mean better. (By all means, place the cost of evaluation on the industry, but let's ensure that the evaluations are conducted on the four issues raised above. There may be squeals from the pharmaceutical industry, but many of the companies are now getting into economic evaluation studies, especially, as in Australia, where they have to get new drugs accepted under the government subsidy scheme.)

One of the biggest advantages of using economic evaluation techniques, beyond the evaluation itself and the promotion of efficiency, is that it encourages decision-makers to think – to think more explicitly about the problem (defining that currently is a major step), to think more comprehensively about possible solutions, to think more coherently about both the advantageous and disadvantageous effects, and to think more lucidly about what weights to attach to these effects, who should do this appropriately, and how. In turn, a second advantage follows from this: if all this process has been gone through before the decision is made, it is far more likely that the decision will be right and can be seen more readily to be right and, consequently and importantly, implemented much more readily. There are powerful forces at work within the health care system, not all of which necessarily subscribe both to the objective of maximising the health of the population in a fair way and to the acceptance of resource constraints. Coherent, systematic decision-making makes it more difficult to get decisions wrong; it also makes it more difficult to attack good decisions on a wrong basis.

On values, as part of evaluation, we need to re-examine medical ethics and in particular the way in which clinical freedom operates in both principle and practice. It is a laudable objective: doing the best one can for one's patients. It is, after all, what the individual consumer's sovereignty often demands. More recognition needs to be taken, however, of the aggregate citizenry's sovereignty. There is a balance here that has to be struck – and struck better than is currently the case.

There can be little doubt that many doctors would suggest that it is their right and duty to defend clinical freedom, believing that if they don't, if they swallow the edicts of economics, then the resources that society will be prepared to devote to health care will fall. In so far as they see themselves able to defend spending on health care, they will attempt to do so. This is very human yet potentially romantic or monotechnic. It is romantic if it is done on the basis of not accepting that there may be an opportunity cost that is greater than the health benefits obtained. It is monotechnic if it accepts the opportunity cost but argues that health is what matters and all other demands on resources are secondary. Beer and cigarettes versus health provides the lexicographic slogan that denies rational thinking – especially at the margin where it matters.

The issue, here, is too important to be left to the doctors. As a society, we have given them the training to allow us efficiently to have medical knowledge available to us. But the medical profession must serve the society that created it. If we educate the profession better, perhaps doctors will better understand the social milieu in which they operate. The final responsibility rests with us as citizens, not with the profession.

Certainly, one place to start is with the way in which clinical freedom operates and is interpreted. One doctor's clinical freedom is another patient's delayed or foregone treatment – or perhaps pint of beer, no matter the financing mechanism. This is more apparent under a public or national health service, although it is there under all health services. How, then, do we reconcile the individual doctor's wish to do the best for their patient, the patient's wish for the doctor to do their best for them and society's wish for an efficient, equitable health care system? How do we embrace not just the individualistic ethics of virtue and duty but also the social ethics of the common good?

First, it needs to be accepted that, by and large, medical ethical codes in concentrating on the individualistic ethics of virtue and duty are correct. Where they go wrong is in their misuse. Consequently, what we need in addition to a medical ethical code is a code of health care ethics.

One, indeed perhaps the primary, advantage of having a code of health care ethics is that it will help to restrict the code of medical ethics to where it belongs: essentially in the world of the individual doctor/individual patient relationship.

But what would such a code look like? To establish that, we need to be more clear as to what its purpose is. Essentially, this would be to try to protect the interests of the community of patients and potential patients (in other words, the aggregate society) in ensuring that good health care is available and accessible and that the proportion of society's resources devoted to health care is well used.

But why do we need such a code? The answer is very similar to the reasons given in Chapter 7 for why we need a medical ethical code. As individual citizens, our knowledge of health and health care in aggregate terms is poor; the search costs involved in finding out more and better are very high. Yet it concerns us that we have good-quality care available to ourselves (remember Margolis' selfish utility from Chapter 8) and accessible to all (Margolis' fair-share notion). But we also want to know that 'our' resources devoted to health care are used efficiently, in terms of both technical efficiency and allocative efficiency. It is in everybody's interest that G', the perceived marginal productivity of the group's resources, is high. A health care ethical code can help to raise G'. Thus, such a code is first and foremost, as was the case for the medical ethical code, for reassurance. The difference is that the former is about reassurance for us as part of the aggregate community, while the latter concerns reassurance for us as individuals qua individuals.

My proposed health care ethical code is as follows:

In order to ensure that good-quality health care is available, all forms of health care that are ineffective should be abandoned.

Subject to legitimate concern about the costs involved in achieving it, the basis of health care should be equal access for equal need.

In order to protect society in the way in which its resources are used in health care, no policy should be pursued that could be pursued by an equally effective but less costly policy.

In order to protect the citizenry's health and the use of their resources, priorities, planning and evaluation in health care should be subject to the principle that only those policies that yield greater benefits than if the resources involved were devoted to some other end should be pursued.

The values on which these decisions should be made ought to be those of society at large; where it proves difficult to elicit these directly, it may be necessary to rely on society's agents to provide the appropriate values. Given their involvement with individual patients, members of the caring professions might have to be excluded from acting as society's agents in these matters.

In other words, my code of health care ethics turns out to be quite simply the rational application of economic evaluation to health care.

To make health care consumption the goal of equity would not be acceptable in most Western democracies; it is too paternalistic. To make health the goal smells of, perhaps, romanticism – and certainly of monotechnicism.

There seems a lot to be said in favour of a health care ethical code.

11.5 Does economic evaluation work?

While the idea of introducing a health care ethical code based on the approach of economic evaluation is very appealing in principle, can it be shown that it might work in practice? Can economic evaluation be made a practical reality?

The extent to which the approach is currently practised in health care is generally quite limited. Of course, much depends on how we define economic evaluation.

It would be depressing, even if perhaps understandable, if we had to conclude that, given the complex and emotive nature of health and health care, decision-making on resource allocation in this sector was inevitably surrounded by less rationality and more prejudice than in any other activity of comparable magnitude. That may be the case, but it is not inevitable.

In a perfect world, with perfect information, the idea of using economic evaluation to maximise the net benefit of health care to society, subject to some concern with equity, is one to which most would subscribe. However, we do not live in a perfect world with perfect information. Consequently, many difficulties arise in attempting to apply the techniques of economic evaluation in health care.

First, while good data regarding health service costs are frequently available, this is less likely to be the case for those costs falling on patients and their relatives and friends.

Second, there is the question of the effectiveness of different types of care regime. Most (but not all) of the practices of medicine produce some improvement in the health state of the patient. It is not for the economist to say how effective various forms of care are. Yet it is unfortunate that the extent to which the medical profession is pressing for improvements in health status measurement (e.g. through QALYs) is all too limited. Certainly the move to EBM in recent years is a step in the right direction. There is, however, a need for care here. No one could be opposed to EBM provided the costs involved in being evidence-based are not too high.

There are dangers, however, in the way in which EBM is currently applied. First, evidence is almost always quantified evidence to the exclusion of other evidence. Second, such evidence seems to concentrate on health alone on the outcome side without first asking what other possible effects might be valued. Third, the question of who to ask about what evidence it is relevant to collect is seldom addressed. There is a risk that the way in which EBM is currently applied leaves us in a world where all that is assumed to be relevant is health and what is given priority is that for which there is quantified evidence.

In June 2000, I attended a basketball tournament in the Pilbara, a remote part of Western Australia. It was run under the auspices of the local public health unit. Organised by Aboriginal health workers as part of a safe sex campaign for Aboriginal youth, it saw 17 teams take part on each of three days and about 500 Aboriginal people attend from the local community on each day. The Aboriginal health workers gained self-esteem from their successful organisation of the event, the teams got good physical exercise, and the local community built community cohesion (and enjoyed themselves). Measurable, evidence-based outcomes? Two broken legs. Yet this programme has to compete for scarce health care resources with dialysis machines.

In essence, the problems of output measurement stem from (1) the multidimensionality of health outputs, (2) the fact that the weightings, whether ordinal or cardinal, are inevitably value-laden, and (3) the fact that there may well be other outcomes (such as information) and even processes (having one's dignity respected) that are valued by patients but that are even more difficult to measure and value than health.

Clearly, and as has been demonstrated earlier in this book, there has been a lot of work in recent years in trying both to develop and to use QALYs in economic evaluation studies. If this work is successful – and some might argue that it is already sufficiently successful to be used – then the problems of achieving multidimensional scaling of outcomes are solved, at least for health. But for some of the other outcomes and processes, it is clear that QALYs cannot cope as, even if valid and reliable measures, they only measure health. Progress is, however, being made in addressing these issues, especially with the use of discrete choice experiments (see, for example, Ryan and Farrar[5]). The problem of valuation arises partly at a methodological level – that is, how do we establish relevant values? – but also, and as a prior issue, at the level of deciding on whose values to apply. This is one of the key questions facing any society in determining resource allocation in health care.

Certainly, this is not an issue that economists themselves can or indeed should attempt to resolve on their own; it involves a social or political judgement. Indeed, this view also incorporates an important moral judgement; that is, it ought not to be within the remit of the economist to exercise their preferences or value judgements for the various states of the world that they are asked to analyse. Despite the moral judgement expressed, it may well be that economists cannot free themselves from this subtle trap.

A third difficulty for the analyst is in trying to influence the processes of resource allocation through the application of economic evaluation. In all health services, the nature of decision-making is diffuse. This would seem to stem from the fact that in health care, perhaps to a greater extent than in any other industry, some of the most powerful workers and most influential decision-makers on resource allocation are, as it were, on the shop floor; that is, the doctors. This results in the chain of decision-making frequently being lengthy and tortuous and embracing the value judgements of many different individuals. (When it is short-circuited 'illegitimately', the problems may be even greater.) An understanding of these administrative, decision-making processes would seem to be a prerequisite for the economist not only wishing to apply economic evaluation to the health care sector but also hoping to influence health care resource allocation. That under-standing has not always been present, at least not in abundance. It can improve and is beginning to improve in health care (see, for example, Jan[6]).

This brief review perhaps goes some way towards explaining why compara-tively few economic evaluation studies have been conducted successfully in health care. Does the rather pessimistic note mean that we should abandon the pursuit of such evaluation in health care and with it our health care ethical code?

Certainly not; the fact that there are problems in practice means two things in essence. First, in attempting to apply economic evaluation techniques we need to be sure that the level of appraisal is appropriate. Second, there is still scope for developing and refining the methodology in the health sector, perhaps particularly in the form of cost–utility analysis.

Let us consider these two issues. First, there is a need to conduct an appraisal of the appraisal itself. We need, for example, to ensure that the objectives of the appraisal are correct. Again, it may be that identifying the costs and enumerating the effects (as opposed to quantifying and valuing the benefits) may on occasion suffice.

Yet again, identifying a series of implied values – that is, the marginal costs in different programmes – for similar types of output (e.g. lives saved) will allow decision-makers to become more consistent in their decision-making and at the same time more efficient. (Thus, if the marginal cost of life saving in one field is £1 million and in another for saving similar lives £100,000, a switch of some resources from the former to the latter will increase the total of lives saved.) Indeed, it may be possible to take this implied-values approach still further and compare dissimilar outputs. Thus, while a greater degree of subjective judgement on the part of the decision-maker would then be required, nonetheless being forced to make explicit the weights they attach to different outputs is likely to create a more efficient decision-making process. There are considerable virtues in pursuing these implied values more systematically and comprehensively and thereafter attempting to generalise from them to allow much more monetary valuation on the benefit side of existing cost-effectiveness studies which, because of this lack, are, in essence, frustrated cost–benefit analyses.

It seems, therefore, that considerable advances can be made using the approach of economic evaluation, without necessarily having to solve all the difficulties discussed above. The main reason for this is that with or without the explicit frame-work and approach of economic evaluation, decisions will be made about resource allocation in health care. The fact that cost–benefit analysis cannot always be applied to health care problems as the purists might wish does not mean that it cannot be an important decision-aiding tool.

Second, there can be little doubt that there remains scope for improving upon the methodology of economic evaluation in the health care sector. Attempting to place monetary values on human life has become almost respectable. Measurement of health has become a major interdisciplinary industry, with economists throwing in their lot with psychologists, operations researchers, sociologists, and many others. The nature of health care production functions is being researched more and more. There is scope for further work; but the current level of activity suggests that some economists, at least, believe that some of these methodological problems are soluble.

Perhaps the best hope for getting an acceptable methodology for economic evaluation in health care rests with cost–utility analysis, and certainly this has advantages over both cost-effectiveness analysis and cost–benefit analysis. Cost-effectiveness analysis is restricted to considering only one form of output, while cost–utility analysis can potentially cope with several dimensions of ill health (including death). Cost–benefit analysis requires, ideally, that all outputs be measured in money terms, whereas cost–utility analysis can stop short of this provided that the relevant outcomes can be contained in QALYs.

It is, in large part, this last proviso that is potentially a problem. QALYs include only health. If there is anything else that patients want from their treatment and care, then it is not included in QALYs. However, the second problem is that cost–utility analysis works only if the opportunity cost of the resources included in the cost per QALY analysis is purely in terms of health or, if you like, QALYs. This immediately means that at best we are restricted to questions of health service resource use, since other social service resource use and patients' and patients' rel-atives' resources, such as time, clearly have opportunity costs that embrace much more than just health. Thus cost–utility analysis at this level cannot get beyond addressing the question (albeit a rather important one) 'How best can we maximise the QALYs from the health service budget?'

These comments do not then mean that we have to abandon cost–utility analy-sis. Rather, there is a need for care in recognising not just the advantages of cost–utility analysis over cost-effectiveness analysis and cost–benefit analysis but also the limitations of the approach embedded in cost–utility analysis. The import-ance of these limitations will of course depend on how cost–utility analysis is used and what questions it is asked to address. It does suggest again, however, that the use of cost–utility analysis to try to assess the most efficient treatment for dealing with a specific health condition is less problematical than its use on allocative effi-ciency questions across health care services more generally.

Perhaps economists have generally been guilty of overselling economic evaluation. A wider recognition of the problems of applying the approach in health care can do nothing but good. It will help to silence the critics, or at least shift the focus of their criticism to more constructive targets. It may also reduce the current tendency for some non-economists to believe that the application of economic evaluation is a simple task. At the same time, it will remind the economist that the tools of economic evaluation are somewhat blunt and in need of sharpening and, in the meantime, cannot be expected to carve out anything other than fairly crude – but nonetheless useful – appraisal apparatus.

What is very clear, however, is that there are insufficient incentives at present to promote efficiency and hence the use of economic evaluation in health care. The very existence of a health care ethical code should help. But other incentives are needed.

11.6 Financing, budgeting and remuneration

I do not want to pursue the general question of financing, although it must be clear that my own preferences lie at the collectivist end of the possible spectrum of financing mechanisms. Those like myself who place substantial weight on the equity goals of health care are likely to share such preferences. (For a review of financing coming to this same conclusion, see Donaldson and Gerard.[7]) Certainly, given a concern for equity, I can see little evidence to support charges, cost-sharing, or whatever we want to call it. There are situations where patients should receive money payments, for example to reduce the transport and travel costs they might otherwise have to bear. (We might even pay them for their waiting time – just think of the impact of this if it came out of the clinician's budget!) There seems little reason to oppose payments to family or neighbour carers, especially where this can be shown to be more cost-effective than professional care.

On financing overall, given the importance that societies currently place not just on health care but on the level of spending on health care, in democratic countries there is a strong argument for having the decision on this lying with the government as the elected representatives of the people. This is clearly not the only way to attempt to control health care spending; it is certainly the most direct, seemingly the most democratic – and potentially the most successful.

Where the key to efficient resource allocation may well lie is in budgeting and in how we pay our doctors. The basic principle on which budgets should be built is that of competence in judging opportunity cost. By this, I mean that a group of surgeons, with others working in the surgical arena and perhaps some lay representatives, are competent to determine such matters as the proportion of the total surgery budget that should go to neurosurgery and whether all the forecast extra monies next year should be devoted to ear, nose and throat (ENT) surgery. An ENT surgeon is not competent to judge whether their call for additional resources should take priority over those of the geriatrician, the community nurse or the physiotherapist.

Frequently, budgeting is seen primarily as a mechanism of control. It is this, but it ought to be seen as fundamental both to rational planning and to economically efficient production functions. A structure of budgets along the lines of Table 11.1 will allow each level of competent decision-makers to plan priorities at their level of awareness.

Budgets would apply at the four different levels; for example, for total health care, for programmes such as the elderly, the mentally ill or surgery, for a sub-programme or specialty such as neurosurgery, and for teams within sub-programmes (such as the neurosurgeon's clinical team in neurosurgery). Those responsible for the total health care of the region or area (politicians and/or the local health board/authority) would decide on the allocation to each programme. Programme management teams would then decide how to allocate their budget across their sub-programmes (e.g. the surgical management team would split the surgery budget across the surgical specialties). Specialty management teams would then allocate their budget to clinical teams within their specialty. In this way, priorities are set and, to a considerable extent, controlled through the budgeting process – at least in so far as resource allocation can be used as a mechanism for pursuing priorities.

At least as important but often less well understood is the role of budgeting in promoting economic efficiency. Left to their own devices and with little or no knowledge of the resources they are consuming, and certainly not of the price attached to them, the individual clinician may well get it right in terms of using the most effective treatments available for those patients they are able to treat. The clinician will, however, almost certainly fall down on economic efficiency, at the level of both minimising resource use for a given output and maximising benefit from the resources available. If clinicians do not know their resource use, how can they minimise it? If the clinician has little control over what types of resources are available (i.e. they cannot substitute nurses for drugs and dressings), then they have no incentive to find out what mix of resources can best serve their patients' interests within some global level of expenditure. Give the clinician a budget and the

Table 11.1 Budget structure

Level 1	Total budget
Level 2	Programme budgets (e.g. care of the elderly)
Level 3	Specialty budgets (e.g. dermatology)
Level 4	Clinical team budget (e.g. clinical team of a neurosurgeon)

responsibility to manage it and the position will change. Whether these advantages of budgeting in principle will work in practice is heavily dependent on getting clinicians both to agree to operate the system and to work out, preferably among themselves, how best to deal with non-compliers. The best mechanism would seem to be to reward those who cooperate (let them have their pet machine) or let Dr Jones deal with the fact that a fellow neurosurgeon's overspending is directly affecting the resources available to Dr Jones' patients. This form of peer review with tightly controlled budgets so that Dr Paul's robbing Dr Peter's patients is there for Dr Peter to see (i.e. opportunity cost is made very visible to the right people) is to be encouraged. Essentially, it means, within surgery, for example, setting the surgeons at each other's throats. It is peer review that might work, since non-compliance hurts and failure to deal with non-compliance in others hurts more.

It is this visibility of opportunity cost, both within a programme and across it into adjoining programmes, that separates budgeting from the issues of cost information. It is the reason why budgeting may work, whereas disseminating cost information alone has seemed inadequate in changing behaviour regarding resource use.

One problem is how to set the budgets in the initial period. One way is to start with last year's spending – but to announce that during the year before you start the process means that everyone will attempt to increase their current spending. Ideally, but it may take time, the budgets should be determined by good medical practice, which in turn should be based on economic appraisal. As a short-run measure, it would seem appropriate in the first year to adopt national average standards (i.e. to allocate out resources on the basis of what the average treatment of, say, a varicose vein operation consists of), or perhaps something just a little below that sum in order to have a contingency fund available to deal with the particularly deserving cases that will inevitably arise in the first year.

Certainly, such budgeting is very desirable if a code of health care ethics is to be translated into a practical management instrument. It is difficult to see otherwise how it will be possible to exercise the necessary control over the clinical freedom fighters.

Beyond the question of budgeting, however, lies the issue of more direct incentives through how we pay our doctors. There is now substantial evidence to show that the way that doctors behave is, in part, a function of how they are paid. (For example, see Krasnik et al.[8])

This is not something that we should lament. Paying doctors for carrying out a particular activity means, *ceteris paribus*, that the probability that they will do it is thereby increased. Paying them still more is likely to increase the probability still more (although the evidence on this latter point is less strong).

Some have argued against fee-for-service medicine. But as a principle, I can see little wrong with it. The basic argument that is used against it seems to be that it will lead to overservicing. It might, but that would seem to depend on two considerations: first, how high are the fees? And second, what is the optimal level of servicing?

If doctors are paid very low fees for some activities, they are unlikely to have any great incentive to carry them out. What a fee schedule could do, if constructed properly, is to encourage some activities and discourage others while, if so wished, the total level of activity of the doctor is held more or less constant. Indeed, one of the advantages of fees is that they can provide differential incentives to help to persuade doctors to pursue some activities more than others.

This is in no sense meant to imply that doctors are then doing something that is ethically or morally wrong in taking account of the relative remuneration in using their time in different ways. Nor is it implying that doctors are just in it for the money. I certainly don't believe that. I am simply suggesting that, given a higher reward for a particular activity, *ceteris paribus*, there is some higher probability that that activity will be conducted.

Second, there is a need to think through what is optimal care in various circumstances. This is where medical audit and clinical budgeting or resource management ought to marry up but seem not to. Best medical practice is efficient medical practice. What we want is some system of incentives to get doctors to practise this optimal level and type of care. But then we have first got to determine what the optimum is. This, to me, is the key to the promotion of efficient health care. Given the nature of the commodity health care, as discussed in Chapter 3, and the agency relationship, as discussed in Chapter 6, the emphasis in health care policy-making on the achievement of efficiency has to be on the medical doctor and not on the patient. The normal rules of demand do not obtain or are, at best, muted in the health care market. It is to the supply side and especially to the doctors that we have to look for the pursuit of efficiency. However, as this does not come naturally to them, they need encouragement; they need sticks and carrots. While finance is only one form of incentive, it can be an important one. There is a need for more experimentation on how best to pay our doctors.

11.7 Listening to the community

What is needed most fundamentally if health care systems are to change and become more socially efficient and equitable is to listen to the informed community voice and to act accordingly. This will do two or possibly three things. It will bolster what is best described as social or community autonomy. It does this ideally not just by allowing the community to have a voice but by permitting the community to be involved and to boost its sense of community. This in turn relates to what was described earlier, communitarianism. This allows us as a society, as a community, to decide in principle the bases on which health care resources should be allocated with what is likely to prove, on the limited evidence to date, a strong weighting to disadvantaged groups and at the same time allowing us to overcome the deficiencies of utilitarian economics, most fundamentally, as Sen has put it, the fact that some people have an inability to manage to desire adequately.

Second, it will move us away from the emphasis in recent health care reforms on a more and more individualistic form of autonomy that has its place very clearly in the market economy. It is doubtful if that can be used as a basis for building an efficient equitable health care system. Here is where choice truly lies – the ideology of individual choice where individuals acting selfishly pursue their own utility and where altruism, if it exists, does so only to foster the utility of the individual who is being altruistic. For example, the only reason I help old ladies across the road is because I feel good, not for their sakes.

Third, the community, given the chance, is likely to be a caring community, or at least it is likely to be more caring than many governments. I am thus advocating listening to the community. We need to do much more eliciting of community values – genuinely community values – and this is not easy. Preferences must be based on constrained choice, and they must be informed.

It is beginning to happen. There is a need for public debate on the values or the principles that we, the community, want to underlie our health service. It is the community's health service; it is not the Health Department's; it is not the Ministry of Health's; it is not the doctors'. This is *our* health service.

Certainly, as an economist, I believe that there is a need for a public debate on the values that are to underpin health care systems and establish the nature of the good that the community wants from its health service. Eliciting community values is also useful in building community autonomy. This is something that is present to a greater degree in other countries and is known in the Scandinavian countries as 'Scandinavian solidarity'.

I debated with others in the *Australian and New Zealand Journal of Public Health* the value base of public health and emphasised there the need, as Jurgen Habermas, the German philosopher, has advocated, for the community to (1) lay siege to the democratic institutions of modern society; (2) recognise that social justice has to lie at the heart of public health, and (3) accept that public health is as much about the public's values as it is about health.[9] We cannot leave all of this to the politicians. They are too distant. We cannot leave it all to the bureaucrats; it is not their job to establish from their perspectives the value base of the health care system. I am confident, however, that most of them would welcome such elicitation from the community.

Bureaucrats have a certain duty, I believe, to be a party to and indeed encourage the elicitation of the community's preferences for health and for health care. Adam Bergson, one of the great minds of welfare economics in the first half of the twentieth century, argued that the main reason for eliciting community preferences was just that: to allow the bureaucrats to know what they ought to be doing, and from what value base they ought to be operating.

No economists or other professionals in the health care field should attempt to drive social values, but we have a certain duty to respect them, certainly to help to elicit them, sometimes even to articulate them.

Academics have certain duties, but the most fundamental I believe is to stimulate thinking and challenging, to encourage debate, to foster learning. Such endeavours again must be led by social values. Whatever we are doing in and around health care, as most readers of this book will be, the point I seek to make is very simple: let us listen to the (informed) voice of the community. Not only will this build social autonomy; it will almost certainly lead to more socially efficient and more equitable health care systems than any alternative route. In terms too of the power relationships within health care decision-making, once the people have spoken ...

11.8 A final thought

It is to be hoped that at least some of the ideas proposed in this book will be welcomed by the medical profession, especially those whose ears are already attuned to the notion of promoting in a just fashion the health of the community at large. Certainly, the ideas have more relevance to a public health care system than a more market-oriented one, although some are common to most health care systems. This is inevitable, since the key to success here is seen in a genuine pursuit of a social cost–social benefit approach to health care, framed in a new code of health care ethics. At present, from my perspective, this is more likely to be achieved through some form of public ownership and public financing.

Much of what I have written may be construed by some of the medical profession as doctor bashing. That is not the intent of this book. For me, the basic issue is clear. We have found the most cost-effective solution to making knowledge of health and health care available to society: we train doctors. Doctors, then, have enormous power to influence the nature of health care delivery whatever the nature of the organisation and its financing. Yet that – the nature of health care delivery, its priorities and its objectives – should be the province of society when it comes to decision-making. Doctors, then, need to be socially controlled. In this process, an increasingly necessary one, economics can help.

All too much to hope for? All too much to hope for from economics, and far too arrogantly ambitious for an economist to claim, under the all too swashbuckling title of *Economics, Medicine and Health Care*, that his discipline can achieve it. But try substituting 'common sense' or 'rationality' for 'economics'; little more than that is claimed in this context. And what then?

Questions

1. What are health care systems about?
2. Who needs educating in health economics?
3. What might a health care ethical code look like?
4. What difficulties are there in using economic evaluation in health care?
5. How can budgeting best be used to promote efficiency?
6. How should we pay doctors?
7. Should we listen to the community?

Notes

1. The description of economics as 'the dismal science' is attributed to Thomas Carlyle in 'On the nigger question' in 1849. T. Carlyle, 'On the nigger question', *Fraser's Magazine for Town and Country*, XL (1849), p 531.
2. World Health Organization, *World Health Report 2000* (WHO Publications: Geneva, 2000).
3. S. Jan, 'An institutionalist approach to health economics', PhD thesis (University of Sydney, 2002).
4. R.G. Evans, 'The dog in the night-time: medical practice variations and health policy', in *The Challenges of Medical Practice Variations*, eds T.F. Andersen and G. Mooney (Macmillan: London, 1990), p 117.
5. M. Ryan and S. Farrar, 'Using conjoint analysis to elicit preferences for health care', *British Medical Journal*, 320 (2000), pp 1530–1533.
6. S. Jan, op. cit.
7. C. Donaldson and K. Gerard, *The Visible Hand: The Economics of Health Care Financing* (Macmillan: London, 1992).
8. A. Krasnik, P. Groenewegen, P. Pedersen, P. Scholten, G. Mooney, A. Gottschau, H. Flierman and M. Damsgaard, 'Changing remuneration systems: effects on activity in general practice', *British Medical Journal*, 300 (1990), p 1698.
9. G. Mooney, 'At the turn of the century which values should drive public health?' *Australian and New Zealand Journal of Public Health*, 24 (2001), pp 111–116.

Index